INTRODUCTION TO HOMOEOPATHIC MEDICINE

Second Edition

Introduction to Homoeopathic Medicine

Hamish W. Boyd
MB, ChB, FRCP(Glas), DCH, FFHom

Second Edition

BEACONSFIELD PUBLISHERS LTD
Beaconsfield, Bucks, England

Second Edition 1989
Reprinted 1997

British Library Cataloguing in Publication Data
Boyd, Hamish W.
 Introduction to homoeopathic medicine. – 2nd ed.
 1. Medicine. Homeopathy
 I. Title
 615.5′32

 ISBN 0–906584–21–3

Phototypeset by Gem Graphics, Trenance, Mawgan Porth, Cornwall in 10 on 12 point Times.
Printed in Great Britain at The Bath Press, Bath.

To my Father, William E. Boyd, MA, MD
a wise physician and a dedicated scientist

Preface to the
Second Edition

In this second edition I have not greatly altered the format of the book. I have however altered the text throughout, in the light of many valuable suggestions and criticisms. In the section on materia medica I have added remedy pictures for Carcinosin, Cimicifuga, Phosphoric Acid, Kali Sulph. and Kali Phos. I have also expanded the 'mentals' in a number of polychrests, adding some of the observations on the essence of remedies from the studies of George Vithoulkas, to whom I wish to express my thanks for permission for their use in this book.

The chapter on research has been revised with the help of Dr David Taylor Reilly, for whose expertise and knowledge I am most grateful.

An appendix of Tyler's *Study of Kent's Repertory* has been added, which I hope will prove useful, as well as some more recent books to the bibliography.

I should particularly like to record my appreciation to the following people, each of whom made a painstaking appraisal of the original book, and whose thoughtful suggestions I have been able to take into account in preparing this new edition: Dr Alastair Jack, Dr David Johnson, Dr Oliver Kennedy, Mr Robert Nichols, the late Dr Robin Pinsent and Ms Anne Saunders.

H.W.B.

Preface to the First Edition

For many years I have felt that we require a textbook of homoeopathic medicine, which includes principles and materia medica in one volume, and which sets down the procedure for case-taking and practical application of remedies. I have attempted in this book to fill such a need.

Apart from some case-taking illustrations, I have purposely omitted descriptions of patients and clinical results, which are excellently presented in books such as Margaret Tyler's *Drug Pictures* and Margery Blackie's *The Patient not the Cure*, and in the older volumes of Kent, Clarke and Nash. This book is not an attempt to convince or convert the sceptic, but to guide the interested doctor in his efforts to understand the basic principles of homoeopathy, and to help him to put these into practice.

In spite of the tremendous advances in scientific knowledge, and their application to our understanding of the workings of the human body in health and disease, there are many who feel that the Art of Medicine has largely disappeared. Suppressing or removing symptoms does not necessarily constitute cure. Cure of a patient is restoring him to a sense of well-being, physical, emotional and mental, which allows him to contribute to the full in his own life and that of the community in which he lives.

Many doctors are concerned about the treatment of their patients with some of our present-day drugs. Other forms of treatment such as hypnosis, acupuncture, herbalism, osteopathy or psychotherapy are now being studied in a search for additional ways of helping people.

Homoeopathic medicine is attracting more and more attention from patients and doctors alike, because they see in it a safe and effective form of treatment, which studies the person as a whole, with particular emphasis on him as an individual. It is not a substitute for conventional medicine, but a system of therapeutics which enlarges and broadens the physician's outlook, and in many situations finds a real cure not possible with our usual drugs.

A good homoeopathic doctor should be a good physician first, and then a knowledgeable homoeopath.

In many situations the patient or doctor is referred to as he or him. This has been done for simplicity, and in most cases could equally well apply to the female sex.

A selection of questions for reflection and discussion are included at the end of the book. These are largely drawn from questions used in the Faculty of Homoeopathy examinations. I hope they will stimulate further reading, and assist doctors who wish to study for this qualification. A glossary of the terms used in homoeopathy is also given at the end of the book, and may prove useful for reference.

I acknowledge with grateful thanks the help I have received from the following persons: the late Dr D. M. Gibson, who gave me permission to use parts of his booklets; Dr Margery Blackie, for all she has taught me over the years, with her vivid descriptions of patients and remedies; Dr R. A. F. Jack, for his help with Accident and Injury Remedies; and Dr R. D. Calcott, for his help with Eye Remedies. I should also like to express my appreciation of valuable comments and criticisms from many colleagues on earlier drafts of the manuscript; in particular from Dr Michael Jenkins, Dr George Burns, Dr Frank Johnson, Dr Anne Clover, Dr Muir Gray and Dr Anne Bennett. I should also like to thank Mrs J. D. MacDonald for her patience in repeatedly typing and retyping the text as alterations and new ideas were added; and John Churchill, my publisher, for guidance and encouragement in preparing this book. We are also indebted to the Scottish Homoeopathic Research and Educational Trust for financial assistance towards publishing.

H.W.B.

Contents

Contents

Contents

Systematic Approach to Materia Medica

Contents

Contents

Materia Medica

Contents

SECTION I

PRINCIPLES AND PRACTICE
OF HOMOEOPATHY

Chapter 1

What is Homoeopathy?

Homoeopathy is a system of therapeutics for treating people and animals on the basis of the simile principle. The word 'homoeopathy' is derived from the Greek words *homoios*, meaning like or similar, and *pathos*, meaning suffering.

> *'Similia similibus curentur.'*
> 'Let like be treated by like.'

But what does this really mean?

In conventional medicine we are taught to think in terms of disease or pathological states, changes from the normal physiological state as a result of outside factors such as infection, trauma or stress, and also conditions arising from allergy or even auto-immunity. In order to treat such disease states we try to make a diagnosis based on symptoms and physical signs. This may enable us to find a cause for which there is a specific treatment or, failing this, to treat the patient's complaints by symptomatic measures.

Although there is now an increasing emphasis on the importance of treating the patient as a whole, medicine in actual fact becomes increasingly fragmented and specialised, and there are few treatments which do affect the patient as a whole.

If we look more closely at our patient we find that, although symptoms of disease fall into a variety of categories which are more or less well-defined, enabling the physician to label the disease or make a diagnosis, there are other symptoms also present. These vary from case to case and are unique to that person. Thus, no one case, even of a well-defined disease like pneumonia, exactly resembles another, any more than two individuals are ever absolutely identical. In other words, the symptoms and signs are modified by the reaction of the patient himself.

When a plant tincture, toxic substance or 'drug' is administered in repeated doses to a group of healthy persons, certain symptoms and signs of toxicity are produced. Some of these are common to many 'drugs', and a few are characteristic of that particular 'drug'. By careful recording it is

1

possible to build up a symptom-complex which is unique to each 'drug'. This is known as a 'proving'.

When the symptom-complex presented by the patient is compared with the symptom-complexes produced by 'drugs', in many cases there will be found a resemblance, often extraordinarily close, between the patient's symptom picture and the picture of the effects of *some* 'drug' on healthy persons.

The basis of homoeopathy is that the most successful remedy for any given occasion will be that one whose symptomatology presents the clearest and closest resemblance to the symptom-complex of the sick person in question. That is: Let like be treated by like.

To give a simple illustration: the effects of peeling an onion are very similar to the symptoms of acute coryza. The remedy prepared from Allium Cepa (the red onion) is used to treat the type of cold in which the symptoms resemble those we get from peeling onions.

The symptoms and signs of acute arsenic poisoning are very similar to the symptoms seen in certain cases of gastroenteritis. Arsenicum is used to treat such cases, not because the patient has taken arsenic, but because the symptoms and signs in the patient are similar to those found in arsenic overdosage.

Whenever we treat a sick person by using a method or a drug which can *cause* a similar picture in other persons, we apply the homoeopathic principle, even if we do it unconsciously.

In conventional medicine we use X-rays and radium, which cause cancer, to treat it also. We use amphetamine in the hyperactive child, although it is normally a stimulant.

Some of the treatments for immunological and allergic reactions are dependent on the use of tissue products or sera derived from infected or sensitised individuals, to produce a response in the patient to that very infection or sensitising agent. Could it be that the 'similar' (or homoeopathy) is used more widely than we realise?

Table 1.1 sets down the two requirements for selecting a similar remedy. On the one hand there is the patient with his clinical history, his personal characteristics and his temperament, and on the other hand there is the 'drug picture' or materia medica. This is made up from our knowledge of toxicology, the symptoms and signs obtained from 'proving' remedies on healthy people, and symptoms added to the materia medica as a result of clinical observation and experience.

So the first and fundamental principle of homoeopathy is the selection and use of the similar remedy.

TABLE 1.1   SELECTION OF THE SIMILAR REMEDY

a) *The Symptom Picture*	b) *The 'Drug' Picture*
Physical characteristics	Toxicology
Local and general symptoms	Provings
Temperament of the patient	Experience

The other, and indeed much more controversial issue, is the use of remedies in what are apparently extremely small quantities. It should be pointed out that this use of what are called *potentised remedies* is an extension of the method evolved by Hahnemann from experiment, and *is not in itself homoeopathy*. The use of the term 'homoeopathic' dose by doctors and scientists, usually in a derogatory or jocular fashion to denote an impossibly small quantity of some drug, is a totally inaccurate use of the term 'homoeopathic', which refers to the simile principle and not to the size of the dose. The method of preparation of remedies is described in Chapter 6, where it will be seen that a potentised remedy is not simply a very dilute solution but a scientifically and accurately prepared remedy.

Homoeopathic practice, however, is not only a question of administering remedies according to the simile principle. In order to do this successfully the homoeopathic physician must develop a different approach to his patient, one which not only seeks to make a diagnosis but also studies the patient as a whole individual, with his or her particular reaction to the causative factors of the illness.

In the course of medical teaching there is often a failure to emphasise that symptoms result not only from causal factors such as trauma, infection, malnutrition and emotional stress, but also from the reaction of the patient's own cells and tissue fluids. The way in which a person reacts to outside factors will vary from case to case, depending on that individual's physical and mental make-up. This explains the puzzling observation that two patients with the same diagnostic label may react in a totally different way, indeed the one may recover and the other die.

The way in which a homoeopathic remedy acts is still not understood, but we should always remember that the recovery of the patient depends just as much on the body's defence mechanism as it does on the drugs we give him – in most cases more so. We know more now about immunity, antibodies, hormonal and autonomic responses, but we still do not know what makes a person feel well. Treatment should not consist merely of removal of symptoms, but in a full restoration of the person's physical, mental and spiritual well-being.

The concept that the stimulus of the remedy triggers off a response which restores biological equilibrium seems a reasonable explanation in the light of clinical observation. This stimulus may be pharmacological at lower potencies, but could be of some other kind, possibly electro-magnetic, in the higher dilutions.

Hahnemann himself considered the action of the remedy to be due to its production of an artificial disease similar to the patient's illness. This artificial disease elicits a reaction from the body, and which in turn cures the illness. The stimulus must be accurate, and the response depends on the initial state of the organism. If the body is sensitive or 'sick' a very small stimulus may be more effective than a powerful material dose.

The aim of homoeopathic treatment is not to remove or suppress symptoms in a specific way, as we often attempt to do in conventional medicine, but to restore the total balance of the organism. The 'totality of symptoms' and their relationship to each other guides us to selection of a remedy which will provide the stimulus to recovery.

The persistence of homoeopathy over the last 180 years, in spite of ridicule and opposition, is proof of its effectiveness in helping sick people, even without as yet a scientific explanation for its action.

Chapter 2

The Origins of Homoeopathy

Homoeopathy was developed and given a scientific basis by Dr Samuel Hahnemann. He was born in Meissen in 1755 and his father was a painter in porcelain. Times were bad but he was determined to be a doctor. He set off for Leipzig at the age of twenty with little money in his pocket, but with the ability to speak eight languages. By means of teaching and translating scientific articles he was able to support himself until he qualified. He then quickly rose to fame, and became known as one of the most distinguished physicians in Germany. However, he saw many faults in medicine as it was then practised and did not fear to make his views known. He saw the insane treated with bodily chastisement and wrote: 'The physician in charge of such unhappy people must have at his command an attitude which inspires respect but also creates confidence.'

The overcrowding, dirt and lack of fresh air in the towns were, he thought, the cause of the epidemics. His plans for isolation hospitals, wider streets and houses with gardens were ahead of his time, and in line with modern teaching. As he practised, he became more and more dissatisfied with the methods of his day, such as bleedings, purgings and blunderbuss prescriptions. He felt that these methods did more harm than good. He decided to give himself to translating scientific literature, even though it meant giving up luxury and living in poverty.

He was asked to translate Cullen's *Materia Medica* into German. Having practised in a swampy district, the prevalent 'fever' was known by Hahnemann to respond to cinchona bark (quinine). Cullen defended the old idea that the action of cinchona on the fever was due to its tonic effect on the stomach. Not so, wrote Hahnemann to Cullen. From practical experience he knew that the strongest mixture of astringents and bitters had no effect on the fever, but that such things as strong coffee, pepper, ignatia bean and arsenic did have some effect. Cullen did not reply, but Hahnemann went on wondering how it did act and decided to take some cinchona bark himself. He was amazed to find that he developed all the symptoms of the 'fever', but without pyrexia. These symptoms disappeared when he stopped taking it. After an interval he tried it again on himself and on some of his family. All produced the same symptoms, varying only in degree. Here was a strange phenomenon; a remedy that was effective for disease, which when given to a healthy person induced the symptoms of that disease. Could there be some natural method of cure here upon which he had stumbled? He went back to the ancient literature and found that Hippocrates and, after him, Paracelsus, mentioned that substances that produced symptoms could also cure them.

Hahnemann now started on his life's work. He gathered a band of willing helpers to whom he gave remedies, and interrogated them daily on any special sensations experienced. He called these 'provings' of the remedy. One remedy was given to a number of 'provers' (healthy persons of both sexes) in repeated daily doses of small quantity and, in later trials, of actual potencies – solutions subjected to serial dilution with shaking (or 'succussion') between each stage. The provers were asked to note in a diary any symptoms and signs they experienced, particularly those which differed from their normal sensations, and symptoms that were strange or unusual. Their reports were discussed and expanded by further questioning, until a very full account was recorded of the symptoms and signs which that remedy could produce.

In this way he built up a materia medica consisting of symptoms that he had experimentally produced in healthy people. This materia medica represented a vast collection of accurate observations. When identified in a sick person, they became the indication of the remedy which, given homoeopathically, would and did bring relief. With this materia medica he started medical practice once more, giving the remedy that had produced the symptoms similar to those of the disease. In its provings, Belladonna had all the signs and symptoms of scarlet fever, so he gave it in an epidemic, with spectacular results. He also found that he had a prophylactic as well as a cure; the one child in a large family who escaped scarlet fever had been taking Belladonna beforehand for some other reason.

In practice, he found that after a small but material dose of the indicated remedy the symptoms were aggravated before any improvement started. However, by diluting and succussing the remedy he found the improvement started with less aggravation. He called this 'potentising', and the process is described in detail in Chapter 6.

After thinking, deducing and experimenting, he presented his views and the results of his labours to the profession:

I believe I have discovered a system which will render the practice of medicine certain and its success brilliant. I have laboured fifteen years to test my discovery – my own experiments and the testimony furnished by the records of medicine convince me of its truth. I lay it and them before you, my colleagues, and I conjure you in the name of truth, in the interest of humanity, to investigate it candidly and without prejudice.

Hahnemann's medical contemporaries reacted with bitter aspersions upon his personal character, contempt and scorn on the system he had unfolded, without a single suggestion to investigate or put it to the test. But having satisfied himself of the value of his discovery he battled on for the rest of his life against opposition from the medical profession, and with an ever-growing number of grateful patients.

In 1812, when the survivors of Napolean's retreat from Moscow drifted back across Europe, they brought the scourge of typhus fever. 'Hahnemann's fame was widespread and he achieved cures bordering on the incredible.' (Hartmann, 1814). He healed 180 cases with only one fatality.

The cholera epidemic invaded Europe eighteen years later, and again his hypothesis was shown to work. One of Hahnemann's pupils had only six deaths among 154 cholera patients. In the same town, of 1500 patients treated by the orthodox methods, 55 per cent died.

Homoeopathy spread to Britain, and there was an attempt by the medical profession to have its practice forbidden by law. A cholera epidemic came to the rescue in 1854. When it was over, the results of treatment in the various hospitals were put before Parliament. Fortunately, a homoeopathic patient was there and asked why those of the homoeopathic hospital had not been included, and demanded that they be procured. They came accompanied by a letter from the Government Inspector. The death rate was 16.4 per cent compared with 51.8 per cent at other hospitals. (These figures are confirmed in the British Museum's records.) He said that they were all true cases of cholera, and he had seen cases recover who would have died in other hospitals. He ended by saying: 'If it should please the Lord to visit me with cholera I would wish to fall into the hands of a homoeopathic physician.'

Hahnemann, having thought through his new methods, published a book called *The Organon*, in which he recorded his thoughts. He had come to the conclusion that there was in man a balancing mechanism which kept him in perfect health, in spite of all the stresses of life (psychological, physical and atmospheric), provided that the stresses were not too great or prolonged, and that the balancing mechanism itself, which he called the 'vital force', was not impaired. But if the stress was too great, or the vital force impaired, unusual signs, sensations and symptoms followed. These were the language of the sick body. The sick body could be restored rapidly to its original state of health by a potentised remedy that had been found by experience to produce a similar condition in a healthy body.

Today a great deal is talked about stress as the cause of ill health, but there is no clear method for treating it. The results of psychological stress are often dealt with by psychiatrists and social workers. To Hahnemann the 'mental symptoms', i.e. those concerned with temperament, emotion, feelings and will, were the most important in guiding him to the correct remedy.

Hippocrates had noticed that 'disease is eliminated through remedies able to produce similar symptoms', but it was left to Hahnemann, nearly 2000 years later, to rediscover this fact for himself, and by a new method of trials on the healthy human being, to develop a new pharmacy and a new method of therapeutics. All over the world this method is still practised by qualified practitioners.

The idea that the body itself might be aided and abetted in its endeavours to cure the disorder and disharmony responsible for disease may have seemed ridiculous and scarcely worthy of attention to the men of Hahnemann's generation. It is by no means so absurd today, with our knowledge of immunology, allergy, molecular biology and even sub-molecular physics. Time and the advance of science are proving to be on Hahnemann's side.

In other respects too, Hahnemann's thinking was ahead of his time. He postulated the theory that disease was in most cases not merely local but systemic, that local symptoms were but outward and visible signs of inward metabolic dysfunction, and that many so-called acute illnesses were but a flare-up or exacerbation of a deep-seated chronic disorder.

In consequence, he argued that in treating an illness it is the whole person who should be considered, and not just the local manifestations of the trouble.

REFERENCES

Samuel Hahnemann: His Life and Work, Richard Hachl.
Homoeopathy, G. Ruthven Mitchell.

Chapter 3

What Does Homoeopathy Offer?

Many people think of homoeopathic treatment as a last resort for difficult or resistant chronic illnesses, where many other forms of treatment have already been tried, but homoeopathy in fact has a wide field of action, especially in primary care and acute illness. Many chronic illnesses can be greatly improved, and advanced disease can be modified or helped to a limited extent – conditions such as severe rheumatoid arthritis or osteoarthritis, motor neurone disease, multiple sclerosis, muscular dystrophy, leukaemias, and certain forms of cancer and severe mental illness. It is still well worth treating these with homoeopathic remedies, selected on an individual basis and taking into account the patient's total symptom picture and mental and physical characteristics, as described later, rather than simply the presenting local symptoms. In this way the disease can be modified, occasionally stopped, and above all the patient's well-being and quality of life can be improved. In cases of cancer, the amount of sedation and analgesia can often be greatly reduced and the patient kept alert and comfortable, even if the ultimate result is the same.

CONDITIONS WHERE CONVENTIONAL TREATMENT IS ESSENTIAL

Surgery

Surgery is essential for removal of mechanical lesions, obstruction, stones, acute appendix, certain inflammatory bowel conditions, tumours and of course repair of congenital defects or orthopaedic problems. In some cases of peptic ulcer, colitis, cholecystitis and renal calculi a homoeopathic remedy will relieve without the need for surgery. Remedies like Arnica, Causticum, Staphysagria and Carbo Veg. can help the patient to recover more quickly and smoothly after surgery.

Deficiencies

Where a patient requires replacement therapy with iron, vitamin B_{12},

9

thyroxine, insulin or hormones, the appropriate treatment with a conventional drug is given in normal dosage.

In gross cardiac and renal failure, and biochemical imbalance, orthodox treatment will usually be necessary, but can be successfully supplemented by homoeopathic remedies.

Severe Infections

In active pulmonary tuberculosis, venereal diseases, meningitis and severe septicaemia, homoeopathic doctors would advocate the use of antibiotics along with homoeopathic remedies.

HOMOEOPATHY IN PRIMARY CARE

In hospital practice, as a young doctor or student, the impression is often gained that we can cure many illnesses and do some dramatic things. It is only when we get out into the field of general practice that we realise many conditions are still very difficult to treat – allergies, skin conditions, rheumatism and arthritis, asthma, migraine, and of course the wide range of psychosomatic illnesses, as well as people who are merely not well.

There is increasing concern on the part of both lay and medical men and women at the amount of illness caused by overprescribing, by side effects and by reactions occurring in sensitive individuals. In general practice, only a small percentage of patients suffer from clear-cut diagnostic disease or conditions which can be treated successfully with all the latest drugs. Doctors who come to study homoeopathy are very often individualists, concerned about the quantity of sedatives, tranquillisers, antispasmodics and antibiotics they are prescribing, and seeking safer and more effective ways of helping their patients. Homoeopathy is not a panacea, but it is of immense value in treating many ailments.

First Aid and Injury

There are a number of useful remedies for accidents and emergencies. These are described more fully in Section II (Chapter 9), the common ones being Aconite, Arnica, Rhus Tox., Calendula, Hypericum and Ledum.

Acute Infections and Respiratory Disease

Although antibiotics have revolutionised acute bacterial infections, the problem of acquired resistance by organisms is well known, and a constant stream of new antibiotics flood the market from the pharmaceutical industry. Side effects can occur with most of these drugs, and others cause allergic reactions in sensitive individuals. The bowel flora is disturbed and fungal infections occur. Antibiotics should be selected with care, and only used if absolutely essential.

Homoeopathic remedies will clear up many sore throats, fevers, coughs and septic lesions without the use of an antibiotic, by helping to stimulate the body's natural defence mechanisms to overcome the infection. They are particularly useful in children with recurring chest infections or tonsillitis, where an antibiotic clears up the acute phase and then relapse occurs within a week or two. Doctors and parents are often concerned at the amount of antibiotics sometimes given to children. They may develop chronic catarrh, secretory otitis media, deafness or discharging ears; their adenoids, tonsils and glands become enlarged and sometimes operation becomes necessary. Homoeopathic remedies can often reduce catarrh, greatly improve the child's health, and avoid these complications. As stated earlier, a remedy is required for that individual child based on his total symptom picture and personality, and not just a local remedy. Chapter 20 on children's remedies describes a number of the useful ones for different types of children, such as Calc. Carb., Pulsatilla, Sulphur and Silica.

In these children, house dust or animal allergy is often the cause of their wheeze or catarrh, rather than an infection. Again, these can be helped by homoeopathic preparations of the allergens, together with appropriate preventive measures against house dust mite.

Influenza
This and certain associated virus diseases, which are virtually unaffected by known orthodox drugs, have responded over the years to the indicated remedy such as Gelsemium, Eupatorium, Rhus Tox., Baptisia and Pyrogen (Chapter 12).

Pneumonia
This was successfully treated by homoeopathy long before the advent of antibiotics. Homoeopathic remedies are still effective, although sometimes an antibiotic is used in addition, in a feeble patient or for a severe infection.

Asthma
This requires careful study to find the causative factors. Some patients may require inhalers or a nebulizer, or in extreme cases steroids, but there are several valuable acute homoeopathic remedies for asthmatic attacks. Even more important, the patient should be treated between attacks by a

constitutional remedy, which will improve his health and reduce the incidence and severity of the attacks, and in many cases completely abolish them.

Gastrointestinal Illness
In Chapter 14 a number of remedies are described which will cure or alleviate acute diarrhoea and vomiting, dyspepsia, peptic ulcer, colitis (particularly irritable bowel syndrome and even some cases of ulcerative colitis), and piles. There are few specifics in homoeopathy, and each case must be individualised to find the best remedy in that situation. The wrong remedy will not work.

Rheumatism and Arthritis
This group of diseases is one of the main causes of disability and loss of working hours. Many of these patients have no obvious pathological change, and merely complain of pain and stiffness, sometimes related to the weather. Homoeopathic remedies will cure these. Where there is advanced bony change and joint damage, the best that can be hoped for is some alleviation and improved mobility. Here again, homoeopathy can do much. It can reduce the amount of analgesics and anti-rheumatic drugs, and often help where the patient cannot tolerate these drugs due to side effects and allergic reactions. Good physiotherapy, occupational therapy and occasionally surgery are also important (Chapter 17).

Headaches
It is essential to exclude severe pathological lesions, like neoplasm or arterial disease, which may require neurosurgery, but the vast majority of headaches are due either to migraine or to psychological stresses and tension. In homoeopathy there are a number of acute headache remedies, selected on the basis of their modalities (factors which modify the pain like heat, cold, pressure, movement, etc.). These are described in Chapter 10.

Even more important, as in asthma, the patient should be treated between attacks with a carefully selected general remedy which suits that individual. In this way the incidence and severity of attacks can be reduced, and in many cases cleared up altogether.

Skin Conditions
It is important to distinguish between external causes of skin disease such as scabies or pediculosis, where a local application will cure the condition, and eczema, dermatitis and psoriasis. These are often skin manifestations of a general underlying problem, due either to heredity, allergies or

emotional stress. Here the homoeopath will try to treat the patient rather than the skin, and will use a minimum of local ointments, especially steroids. The concept of suppression of skin disease resulting in more deep-seated internal illness is discussed elsewhere (pages 31 and 32); many doctors have observed an eczema or dermatitis apparently clearing up with local applications, but in fact being suppressed, and being followed by asthma or gastric symptoms.

Remedies for shingles are also discussed in the section on skin. Rhus Tox. and Ranunculus Bulb. will often act very quickly, relieving the burning pain and encouraging rapid healing (Chapter 16).

Genito-urinary Disease

Although a large or impacted calculus may require surgery, the remedy Berberis will often relieve the pain of renal colic and encourage passage of a stone. Acute cystitis may on occasions require an antibiotic, especially in younger patients where there is proven bacterial infection, but remedies like Cantharis, Causticum and Terebinth are often all that is required. The problem of recurring attacks of cystitis or chronic infection is a difficult one in practice, and here the homoeopathic remedy for the patient, or a bowel nosode like Sycotic Co., is often of value. Prescribing in this way will reduce the need for repeated antibiotics and, in some patients, stop the relapses entirely.

There are a number of remedies for the treatment of leucorrhoea, dysmenorrhoea and the symptoms of the menopause, but these should be selected for the individual patient based on her general and mental symptoms, and not merely on the local pain or discharge. Where there is a large fibroid or ovarian cyst, or an obvious prolapse, surgery will be necessary (Chapter 15).

Cardiovascular Disease

Where a patient has cardiac irregularities or gross heart failure, drugs like digoxin or diuretics may be necessary, and in acute myocardial infarction intensive care may be required; but there are many valuable remedies in homoeopathy for angina and heart failure, such as Crataegus, Cactus, Carbo Veg. and Lachesis. Patients with hypertension should always be given a remedy based on their total symptomatology, as well as local organ remedies, before resorting to diuretics, beta-blocking drugs or other anti-hypertensive agents, particularly if they are elderly.

In cases of cerebrovascular accident, remedies like Arnica, Opium and Gelsemium can sometimes bring about remarkable improvement (Chapter 13).

Psychosomatic Illness and Anxiety States

In general practice there are a large number of patients who present with illness resulting from stress, emotional upsets or environmental situations, and these may cause nervous symptoms or even physical signs. It is important to find the underlying cause of a patient's stress or anxiety, by gentle questioning and listening. If this can be helped or resolved, a homoeopathic remedy can be of great assistance in restoring the patient to well-being and health. It will be seen that the homoeopathic method of case-taking, with its detail and emphasis on emotional symptoms, may well play a valuable psychological part in aiding recovery, although this should be a part of all medical history-taking if time allows. While there is an awareness of the need for preventive medicine, and of a positive attitude to health as opposed to disease, there is often no suitable orthodox remedy which can be prescribed before pathological changes have started. Homoeopathic remedies can deal with illness in its early stages, and perhaps prevent the development of more serious disease.

Only a brief summary has been given in this survey of possible fields of use for homoeopathy. There is almost no situation in which a homoeopathic remedy is not of some value, except perhaps in some instances where the patient is receiving intensive medication with several potent conventional drugs.

The homoeopathic doctor is always searching for a more effective remedy, and a fuller understanding of his patient and that person's need. Every patient is an individual problem, with his own unique personality and reaction, and not just 'a case of bronchitis or colitis'. It is perfectly possible to combine homoeopathy with conventional medicine in many situations, but with increasing experience the doctor will find himself using less of the palliative drugs, and more homoeopathy, with the satisfaction of curing his patients in the true sense.

It should be stated firmly that homoeopathy does not consist of using conventional drugs in inadequate dosage. Where a conventional drug, analgesic, sedative, antibiotic or cardiac drug is used by a homoeopathic doctor, it is used in the correct orthodox dose. Only homoeopathic potencies are given in their specially prepared dilutions.

In Section II remedies are grouped under the body systems, with descriptions of the leading symptoms for each remedy on which to prescribe. Some doctors will find these a useful starting point for prescribing, until they have grasped the concept of remedies for 'people' rather than for 'diseases'.

Chapter 4

The Materia Medica

Mention was made in Chapter 2 of the 'proving' of remedies, the method whereby symptoms and signs of minor or major toxicity, from administering repeated small doses of a substance to healthy volunteers, were collected and assessed.

This 'proving' has continued over the years, using a wide variety of substances. Tinctures of plants, salts, metals, venoms of snakes and spiders, and even certain synthetic drugs have all been 'proved', and their symptoms and signs recorded and assessed. In addition, the known toxicology of each substance has been added. A third group of symptoms and signs – those which have been helped or cured by the particular remedy in a reasonable number of patients – have also been included.

These three groups make up the detailed materia medica used by the homoeopathic physician. They form the symptom-complex characteristic of the remedy (see Table 1.1, page 3).

1) Poisoning and toxicology.
2) Provings.
3) Experiential symptoms.

In addition to these factual records, observations have enabled physicians to associate certain characteristics of appearance and temperament with the effectiveness of particular remedies. This makes it possible to select a suitable remedy for the patient by taking into account his whole physical and mental make-up, in addition to the detailed analysis of his symptoms.

A drug has a certain chemical composition, causes particular effects on body physiology or pathology, and is used for a specific purpose or disease. However, every drug also produces side effects or toxic reactions, and it is these which the homoeopathic doctor takes note of and uses as a part of his materia medica. Most of the remedies used in homoeopathy are derived from *naturally* occurring substances – whole plants, minerals and salts – and not from single extracts or refined synthetic products. This does not mean that a 'pure' synthetic drug cannot be used homoeopathically, but a

15

fresh 'proving' would have to be carried out to find the 'drug picture' of that substance. It is for this reason that we retain the Latin name for a remedy, such as Natrum Muriaticum, instead of calling it Sodium Chloride, which would infer a purified product. The source of Natrum Mur. is described in the pharmacopoeia, and the remedy of that name is known throughout the world in any language.

THE REMEDY PICTURE

Each remedy in the materia medica contains a description of the symptoms and signs associated with it, set out under the systems of the body. These vary from apparently minor symptoms to gross toxic effects, the amount of detail depending on the text. One of the characteristic features of a homoeopathic materia medica is the inclusion of modalities of symptoms. These are things which qualify a symptom – for example the type of pain and what things make it better or worse: movement, rest, heat, cold, damp, time of day. In addition to local symptoms, we find general symptoms affecting the person as a whole, and mental symptoms related to the temperament, emotions and feelings. It is necessary in studying a remedy to memorise as much as possible of the characteristics of that particular remedy, and the organs it affects, and also to note if there is one kind of symptom running through the various systems. For example, in Bryonia we find marked dryness and aggravation from movement appearing in many local areas, or cramping pains in Cuprum, or stitching pains in Kali Carb.

Examples of prominent features in certain remedies are:

Aconitum: Acuteness of onset, extreme restlessness, marked fear, intense thirst.
Belladonna: Bright red face, bounding pulse, burning hot skin, staring eyes with widely dilated pupils, an aggressive type of delirium.
Sulphur: Widespread burnings, disturbances of circulation, marked intolerance of heat.

A similar set of symptoms can be found in patients, and the details of this are explained in the next chapter on case-taking. It is the matching of these two sets of symptoms in patient and remedy which is the essence of homoeopathic prescribing; in other words, the selection of the similar remedy.

Because of the great number of remedies and symptoms, doctors using homoeopathy have compiled dictionaries or 'repertories'. These show what symptoms are present in different remedies, and indicate their importance. The best known repertories are those of Kent, Boenning-hausen, Boericke and Clarke, and more recently the *Synthetic Repertory* of Barthel and Klunker. Card repertories are now in use by Kishore and Brousallian and Flury, and the information from many of these is being put on computer, with a view to simplifying remedy selection.

In using a repertory it is necessary to take a careful case history, to select the symptoms which are most prominent, along with their modalities, and then to look these up under the system affected, e.g. general, mind, extremities, stomach, cough, bladder, etc. Here you will find symptoms described in the patient's words and then a number of remedies in different typefaces. The remedies in heaviest type are the most important to consider. By studying a number of symptoms, certain remedies will be seen to come through strongly, and these should be studied further in the materia medica to obtain the best selected remedy. A description of how to study Kent's *Repertory* is given as an Appendix.

Whilst it is of obvious interest to know the origin of the remedy, it is also helpful from the point of view of treatment, for remedies fall into groups – botanical, chemical, biological – and members of a group are often complementary in action. They will follow each other well, and indeed enhance the effect.

This does not mean that they are interchangeable, for it is usually just one remedy that is eminently suited to the needs of the patient. But one member of the group may act synergistically with another, and it sometimes requires more than one remedy in series to bring about the desired cure.

Next, the pharmacology of the remedy and its sources is worthy of study. It reveals affinities with particular tissues, organs or systems that render the symptoms associated with the remedy more understandable. The knowledge of these tissue or organ affinities may also be of value in prescribing. Examples are the known affinity of:

Iodum with the thyroid gland,
Chelidonium with the liver and gallbladder,
Belladonna with the central nervous system,
Cantharis with the genito-urinary system,
Rhus Toxicodendron with the locomotor system,
Ruta Graveolens with the periosteum,
Arnica with injured tissues,
Hypericum with nervous tissue,
Sepia with the female pelvic organs.

17

Awareness of these tissue affinities may suggest the possible use of one or more remedies, which can then be studied for suitability with other features of the individual case.

Homoeopathy studies and deals with the individual as a whole. The individual remedy must be approached, understood and known in the same way. The remedy picture must be seen as a whole with its own individual features, so distinctive as to be recognised promptly when its counterpart is met in a sick person. This can only be acquired by continual study, coupled with constant observation.

REFERENCES

Materia Medica Pura, Samuel Hahnemann.
Dictionary of Practical Materia Medica, J. H. Clarke.
Materia Medica with Repertory, W. Boericke.
Lectures on Homoeopathic Materia Medica, J. T. Kent.
Keynotes of Leading Remedies, M. C. Allen.
Homoeopathic Drug Pictures, M. L. Tyler.
Condensed Materia Medica, C. Hering.
Studies of Homoeopathic Remedies, D. M. Gibson.

REPERTORIES

Repertory of Homoeopathic Materia Medica, J. T. Kent.
Boenninghausen's Characteristics and Repertory, Translated by C. M. Boger.
Clinical Repertory, J. H. Clarke.
Practical Repertory, R. Flury.
Synthetic Repertory, H. Barthel and W. Klunker.

Chapter 5

Case-Taking and Diagnosis

In many ways case-taking for the homoeopathic physician is different from that of his orthodox colleagues. He must not only make a diagnosis in the usual way, where this is possible, but he must also be thinking at the same time of a suitable homoeopathic remedy, based on the patient's own characteristic reaction and symptom picture.

Accurate and painstaking history-taking is at the very heart of the homoeopathic approach. Only by this can the all-important details of the particular illness and the individual characteristics of the particular patient be arrived at, matters essential for the selection of the similar remedy.

In the first place, every effort should be made to discover as far as possible what is going on, and what is going wrong, in the body of the sick person: what organs are diseased, what functions are deranged, what tissues are damaged or disordered.

These are pertinent questions, and the answers to them, when available, may reveal a need for surgical, dietetic, supportive or substitutionary treatment. A diagnosis must be made, wherever possible. Nevertheless, the risk of being over-engrossed in the 'part' to the neglect of the 'whole' must always be borne in mind.

Knowledge of underlying pathology, in addition possibly to pointing to the need for surgical or other ancillary measures, may be of assistance to the homoeopath because of his knowledge of 'tissue affinities' (Chapter 4). The relation of certain remedies to specific organs or tissues may be of significance for therapy, when such organs or tissues are known to be involved in the disease process.

A careful *physical examination* must always be carried out after history-taking. The full facilities of modern diagnostic techniques should be utilised, when these are relevant and in the genuine interests of the patient.

19

ACUTE CASE-TAKING

When presented with an acute illness, the doctor should try to select a few outstanding symptoms and signs presented by the patient, study the modalities of these and take into account the appearance and immediate mental symptoms of the patient, in particular any change from the patient's usual temperament. This will become clearer when you study the Materia Medica in relation to acute illnesses. Such things as restlessness, fear, irritability in a normally placid individual, desire for company or wish to be left alone, thirst or its absence in a fever, as well as the modalities of the cough or pain, will enable selection of a remedy to be made rapidly with the minimum of questioning (See Table 5.1, page 33).

In young children, the observations of the mother or nurse will be of particular value.

CHRONIC CASE-TAKING

The Complaint and Present History
Attention must first be paid to the particular symptoms of which the patient complains, both in relation to the present illness and also any other troubles. The latter may be considered of minor importance by the patient, but may well be of signal significance in remedy selection.

Onset and Course of the Illness
A sudden onset and rapid development may point to Aconitum or Belladonna. Insidious onset and gradual progress suggest Bryonia, Gelsemium or Pulsatilla.

Enquiry must include any possible *cause* of illness, either recent or remote. The aetiological factor can be of considerable importance in pointing to a definite remedy.

A history of illness coming on quickly after exposure to severe dry cold would suggest Aconitum, Hepar Sulph. or Causticum; illness ensuing after getting chilled when hot, or after a soaking with rain, might require Dulcamara; effects of loss of sleep might point to Cocculus; a history of head injury, perhaps remote, would suggest Natrum Sulphuricum or Arnica. Aconitum may also be indicated where the history of onset dates from a bad fright or shock.

Again, the character of the pain or other symptoms must be enquired into, the sort of pain, the site, the spread, the severity and, above all, the modalities.

20

Modalities

A modality is something which qualifies a symptom and often enables a choice to be made between two quite strongly indicated remedies. These may be of various kinds:

Thermal modalities relate to reactions to heat and cold. Heat may aggravate or give relief, cold likewise. These effects are highly characteristic of individual remedies.

Meteorological modalities are of great importance – the effects of weather changes, wet, wind, thunder, sea air and the like.

Physical modalities such as the effects of rest, posture, active movement, passive movement, exertion, jolt or jar.

Time modalities refer to aggravation or relief of symptoms at a particular hour of the day or season of the year.

A further aspect sometimes comes into consideration, namely laterality. It so happens that many remedies show a relation to symptoms which are predominantly either right-sided or left-sided, or spread in a characteristic manner. For instance:

Symptoms starting on the right side and spreading to the left point to Lycopodium; those starting on the left and extending to the right suggest Lachesis; symptoms which shuttle from side to side point to Lac Caninum; pain shooting centrally up a limb points to Hypericum; pain shooting down the limb suggests Kalmia; pain spreading in all directions points to Dioscorea.

Past History

A history of such illnesses as asthma, eczema, hay fever, rheumatic fever, pleurisy, kidney disease, tuberculosis or venereal disease, or of previous operations, is of course relevant. To the homoeopathic physician a history of injury might call for Arnica, severe reaction to smallpox vaccination might indicate the need for Thuja, or a history of never having been well since measles would suggest the use of Morbillinum.

Family History

Knowledge of the health of parents and siblings can be helpful, not only on account of inherited illnesses, but because a history of cancer or tuberculosis might well indicate the need for Carcinosin or Tuberculinum in the patient.

Having obtained details of the patient's complaint and present history, the past and family history, we must then obtain details which will tell us more about the patient himself, his reactions and temperament. These can be classified under certain main headings.

Physical Characteristics
Both provings and clinical observations have shown a close relationship between remedies and outstanding physical features – complexion, appearance, manner, colour, peculiarities of hair, skin, discharge, movements, posture, speech and odour.

Features which stand out are at once connected by the observer who knows his materia medica with a remedy which has the same features prominent in its drug picture. For example:

The tense, well-groomed, fastidious Arsenicum patient, unable to relax or stay put even at night.
The pale, podgy, phlegmatic chilly Calcarea patient.
The tall, delicate-looking, red-haired Phosphorus patient, fidgety, and nervously anxious to assist and give accurate answers when questioned.
The stoop-shouldered, rather unkempt, red-faced talkative, self-opinionated, warm-blooded Sulphur patient.

It should be pointed out, however, that although these characteristic features may help in selecting a remedy, not every tense well-groomed person is Arsenicum, nor every red-haired patient a Phosphorus. These are merely additional guides to remedy selection.

General Physical Symptoms
These refer to the patient as a whole, and may be features which the patient exhibits even while in perfect health. However, if the patient's response differs from his normal this is more significant and should be noted. Effects in general of bathing, wetting, pressure, rubbing, jarring, defaecating, can be useful to elicit.

Temperature
Effects of temperature on the person as a whole. Nux Vomica types are excessively chilly, and hug the fire in winter. Pulsatilla persons on the other hand dislike hot weather, are ill at ease in a hot stuffy atmosphere, crave air and want windows widely open, get overheated in bed and push off the covers, but may before long feel chilly and pull them on again. Remember a person may feel the cold but dislike stuffy atmosphere (better in fresh air). He may be worse from heat in general but better with heat locally – for example Lycopodium, in whom heat to the stomach or rheumatism helps, but general heat aggravates; Secale who likes heat for headache or neuralgia but is generally worse from heat, or Phosphorus

who is worse from cold but likes cold drinks and cold applications or cool air for the headache.

Weather

This has been mentioned under modalities, but may also affect the patient as a whole, in which case it becomes a general symptom. Does he feel worse or better in damp, cold, frost, windy, stormy or thundery weather, or at the sea?

In rheumatism we expect as a rule to have an aggravation from weather changes, on the joints or muscles or on the person's wellbeing. The absence of such an aggravation becomes peculiar and characteristic, and allows us to exclude certain remedies. If *change* of weather does not affect rheumatism, we can exclude Dulcamara, Nux Moschata, Phosphorus, Ranunculus Bulbosus, Rhododendron, Rhus Tox., Silica, Tuberculinum; or if *wet* weather does not affect it we can eliminate Calc. Carb., Mercurius, Natrum Carb., Natrum Sulph., and Ruta.

Absence of particular symptoms that strongly characterise a remedy cannot be relied on as excluding that medicine, yet when strong general symptoms that characterise the remedy are absent we can, with a fair degree of confidence, exclude that remedy.

Perspiration

Does he perspire and if so where – head, feet, body? Head sweats at night, soaking the pillow, suggest Calcarea Carb. Sweaty malodorous feet could indicate Silica. General perspiration at night might indicate Tuberculinum, and especially if without relief, Mercurius. Sometimes the sequence of events in chill, fever and perspiration may be significant.

Time

Many patients appear to have an aggravation of their symptoms at particular times of the day or night. If this aggravation is of a recurrent nature, for example the cough or fever is always worse in the evening, or the patient feels generally worse at that time, this may provide specific indications for the selection of the correct remedy. Some well-known times of aggravation are 1–2 a.m. (Arsenicum Album), 3–4 a.m. (Kali Carb.), 4–8 p.m. (Lycopodium). Morning aggravation may suggest Chelidonium, Natrum Mur. or Nux Vomica. Evening aggravation possibly indicates Bryonia, Pulsatilla or Belladonna. Periodic return of symptoms may be significant in an illness *not* characteristically of a periodic kind in its pathology (not so valuable an indication in malaria). Alternate days might suggest Chininum Sulph. or Lycopodium; every two weeks, Arsenicum Alb. or Lachesis.

Position

The influence of this on the patient as a whole is a general symptom. Aggravation by standing of Sulphur or Valerian, aggravation kneeling of Sepia, aggravation lying on the right side of Mercurius, the peculiar aggravation of Phosphorus when lying on the left side, and yet aggravation of head symptoms when lying on the right.

Senses

Sensitivity to noise, light, smells (nausea at the smell of cooking, or thought of food), travel sickness.

Food Cravings and Aversions

These are only of value if they are strong likes or dislikes and are not influenced by advice, habit, religion or other factors.

The commonest helpful ones are desire for or aversion to sweet food, sugar itself, salt, highly seasoned food, eggs, fat, milk, fish. This should be distinguished from foods which upset although desired.

Peculiarities of appetite are associated with many remedies. Natrum Muriaticum subjects are proverbially hungry, eat heartily but remain thin. Several remedies, notably Phosphorus and Sulphur, show a mid-morning empty sensation which demands a snack for relief.

Lycopodium subjects have very capricious appetites; they may feel quite hungry immediately after a meal or they may feel full after only a few mouthfuls. Desire for such things as chalk or coal suggest Calcarea Carbonica.

Food likes and dislikes vary a great deal from one person to another. Lycopodium subjects have a great preference for hot meals and very hot fluids. Phosphorus types, on the other hand, want spicy food, cold meals and even ice-cold drinks. A craving for salt strongly points to Natrum Muriaticum. Food intolerances are many, and if marked in the individual may have their counterpart under one or more remedies. When taken into account with other features in the case, all these personal peculiarities assist in arriving at and choosing a remedy that is most suitable because it is most similar on several counts.

Thirst is another aspect of some significance. Some remedies, notably Apis, Gelsemium and Pulsatilla, show absence of thirst in situations when this would not be expected, i.e. in acute pyrexia. Natrum Muriaticum subjects are usually extremely thirsty.

A desire for frequent sips of water points to Arsenicum Album. A demand for large amounts at long intervals suggests Bryonia. Excessive thirst associated with a poor appetite points to Sulphur.

A general feeling of improvement or aggravation from eating, or its effect on parts other than the stomach, e.g. pains in the limbs ameliorated by eating (Natrum Carb., Kali Bich.) can be classed as a general symptom.

Sleep

The pattern of sleep, position in sleep, and the type of dreams may be of value. Some patients lie awake for hours, others will sleep and then wake at 1.00 a.m. (Arsenicum Album), or 3–4 a.m. (Kali Carb.) The Pulsatilla child often sleeps with his hands above his head. The knee-elbow position may indicate Phosophorus or Medorrhinum. A Lachesis patient cannot bear to lie on the left side, because her heart beats strongly. Dreams may be recurring and of significance – of fire, the dead, escaping, etc. The repertory will often indicate remedies with these marked symptoms. Some remedies have the symptoms 'relief from sleep' (Phosphorus, Sepia) or 'aggravation from sleep' (Lachesis, Sulphur) or effects of loss of sleep (Cocculus).

Menstrual Disturbances

The effect of the period on the patient's well-being as a whole is a general symptom, e.g. worse before and relieved by the flow, or worse during or after menses. Variations in the appearance of the flow, type of pain and of discharge are particular symptoms, but a general irregularity, or profuse or scanty flow, may be classified as a general symptom.

Alterations in sexual desire may be important, either increase or loss of libido, tendency to masturbation, impotence or frigidity.

Mental Symptoms

In selecting the correct homoeopathy remedy these symptoms rank highest in importance. The patient's personality, temperament and psychological features may be assessed to some extent by observation. Questioning may elicit such things as fears, attitude to heights or enclosed spaces, tidiness or the reverse, irritability, weepiness, a like or dislike of sympathy or of company, a tendency to worry or become extremely upset in anticipation, sensitivity to noise and also hobbies and interests.

It is, however, the deviation from the normal that is most important – in what way is the patient different from usual. There are three groups of mental symptoms to be studied in the patient, and in order of importance they are those pertaining to the *Will*, the *Understanding* and the *Memory*.

Will

These include symptoms like quarrelsome, angry, irritable, tearful, hate of loved ones, fearful, intolerant of sympathy, tendency to curse, contrariness, cowardice, hatred, jealousy, suspicion, loquacity, indifference, sadness. Ailments from anger, grief, bad news, love, joy, reproach or resentment, sexual excesses.

This group is of most significance.

Understanding

Delusions, hallucinations, illusions, delirium, loss of sense of proportion, clairvoyance, dullness, difficult or easy comprehension, excitement, mental disability, ailments from mental exertion.

Memory

Absent-minded, error in answers, mistakes in speech and writing, disorders of speech.

Mental Characteristics

In these days the importance of the psychogenic aspect of disease is being realised more and more. From its inception homoeopathy has always emphasised the significance of the mental, especially the emotional features in a case history. Many remedies are intimately related to outstanding psychological symptoms. For example:

The utter apathy and indifference of Sepia.
The jealousy of Lachesis.
The abysmal suicidal gloom of Aurum Metallicum.
The tiresomely fussy tidiness of Arsenicum.
The nervous apprehension before an ordeal of Argentum Nitricum.
The emotional instability of Ignatia.
The disdainful superiority of Platina.
The tearfulness and variability of Pulsatilla.
The intractable irritability of Chamomilla.

This whole range of temperament and mental attitudes, sensitivities and even odd sensations, as recorded under different remedies, affords pertinent pointers to their use.

With experience, the doctor will learn to assess many aspects of a patient's temperament and personality merely by observing how he or she responds to questioning, the way he behaves or his mannerisms in the home or consulting room, without actually asking specific questions. He will sense whether he is outgoing and extrovert, or only giving very guarded answers. He will see if he is tearful or resentful, irritable or tidy, and in this way form a picture of the patient as a person, and hence what remedy may suit him.

Particular Symptoms
These are symptoms related to parts, and may well have been obtained in the present history. It is important to enquire about the modalities in relation to particular symptoms, i.e. the factors which qualify a symptom, as described on page 21.

Common Symptoms
These are symptoms common to many illnesses and to many patients, and are therefore of little use in selecting a remedy, although a common symptom with a *peculiar modality* may be of value, e.g. chilliness in bed, before urination, stool, menses, eating. Weakness while eating, before a storm, after stool. The chilliness of Pulsatilla, worse when near a fire, or the special localisation of a common symptom, the aching pain at the inferior angle of the right scapula found in Chelidonium.

Two common particulars occurring together may be significant, e.g. coryza and polyuria (Calc. Carb.).

Strange, Rare and Peculiar Symptoms
This term in homoeopathic literature is used to include inexplicable reactions. For example: asthma relieved by lying down; difficulty in swallowing liquids, whereas solids present no problem; symptoms with laterality or time aggravations.

Any symptom which is unusual, and especially not explicable in pathological terms but rather characteristic of the patient himself, whether general or local, may be classed as a strange, rare and peculiar symptom. These symptoms are particularly valuable in trying to select a remedy, and will often outweigh many other symptoms.

Observation
During the taking of the patient's case history, which should be obtained with as little interruption as possible, certain observations can be made, which may greatly facilitate selection of the remedy.

Posture
A patient sitting tense and erect on the edge of the chair suggests Arsenicum Album. One who flops into the chair and lounges at full length, omitting perhaps to remove his hat, might point to Sulphur. One who sits

there wringing her hands, probably Ignatia or Phosphorus. One with constant movements, especially of the feet, suggests the possibility of Zincum Metallicum.

Manners
Excitement suggests Phosphorus; apathy points to Sepia; obviously holding back tears, likely to be Natrum Muriaticum; haughty and disdainful, Platina.

Complexion
Bright red face points to Belladonna; quick changes of colour would suggest Ignatia; pallor of lips, ears and fingers would indicate Calcarea Carbonica.

Expression
A scared panicky look points to Aconitum; a furtive glint in the eye suggests Lachesis; a bashful, bored appearance may indicate Baryta Carbonica; a deep furrow above the root of the nose typifies Lycopodium.

Hair
Dry, lustreless hair would suggest several remedies, among them Medorrhinum and Psorinum; sleek well-kept hair might point to Arsenicum Album; alopecia areata would suggest Phosphorus; strikingly red lips would point to Tuberculinum.

Speech
This is especially worthy of note. A spate of words, uttered rather disjointedly, jumping from subject to subject, points to Lachesis; pontificating coversation in the manner of the club bore strongly suggests Sulphur; readiness to reply, with perhaps some hesitation for the sake of accuracy, indicates Phosphorus.

Clothes
May suggest Arsenicum Album if strikingly smart and neat; the reverse, a somewhat untidy, unkempt look would point to Sulphur.

Odour
An offensive body odour would suggest Mercurius or Psorinum; a sour smell of discharges or stools would point to Calcarea Carbonica; a pungent cadaverous odour would suggest Baptisia; a particularly foul odour would point to Carbo Vegetabilis or Psorinum.

The remedies mentioned are just a few examples from the materia medica. (See also Table 5.2, pages 34–5.)

Having taken the patient's history and examined him or her, the prescriber has several choices. He may prescribe:

1) A *Specific Remedy* (e.g. Arnica for the effects of injury, Berberis for renal colic) without taking into account the more general and mental aspects of the case.
2) A *Local* or *Organ Remedy*. This is usually based on the pathology of the case or a local complaint, and requires modalities of symptoms in order to select the remedy. This will usually be prescribed in low potency twice daily for long periods.
3) A *Fundamental* or *Constitutional Remedy*. This prescription is made as a result of assessing the whole symptom picture based on the case-taking just described.

In a busy practice or clinic, the prescriber may use 'keynotes' to select a remedy – three or four characteristic, dominant symptoms which feature strongly also in a remedy.

THE CONSTITUTIONAL REMEDY AND THE FUNDAMENTAL REMEDY

These terms lead to confusion amongst those studying homoeopathy, and indeed many experienced homoeopaths use the terms in rather differing ways.

Professor Dorcsi and Gerhard Koehler describe 'Constitution' as the inherited and acquired physical, emotional and intellectual make-up of a person. It reveals itself in the habit, the basic emotional and intellectual inclinations, and the way the individual reacts to internal and external stress factors.

Dispositions and diatheses develop on the basis of different potentials for illness inherent in the constitution.

Recently some prescribers, notably Professor Eizayaga, have started using the term 'constitution' to describe the normal make-up of the person. They prescribe a 'constitutional' remedy based on this normal picture as a prophylactic remedy to enhance resistance. In treating disease they use the 'fundamental' remedy. This is based on the total presenting symptom picture, especially changes from the normal, and incorporates the pathological symptoms as well as the general and mental symptoms. In some situations the constitutional and the fundamental remedies will be one and the same, and in others they will be different.

In chronic illness we therefore have to look further than the presenting symptom picture and bear in mind the past effects of heredity, previous illness and environmental influences.

We have discussed the need, wherever possible, and in particular in chronic disease, to look at the whole patient. To seek symptoms referable not just to his complaint or the particular part of the body, but also to his general reactions to weather and food, as well as seeking his mental symptoms. In this way we use the totality of symptoms to select a remedy.

Following Hahnemann, other homoeopaths, especially Kent in America and Margaret Tyler in Britain, began to introduce a further concept. This was the idea that people of a certain build, colouring or appearance, with certain distinguishable characteristics of behaviour or mannerisms, and of a certain temperament, seemed to respond to particular 'polychrest' remedies (certain frequently-used remedies with a wide spectrum of clinical symptoms). So, in addition to taking the actual presenting symptoms, they learned to observe and assess their patients as individuals of a particular type. We have already made comments about the Arsenic, Sulphur or Pulsatilla type. The remedy was then often selected on the basis of the patient's type. This is noticeable in Borland's descriptions of children, described in Chapter 20. The concept of constitutional types has become a part of homoeopathic prescribing, although in fact it is not an original Hahnemannian idea.

Constitutional prescribing is of value in the early stages of disease, and particularly after an acute episode. It seems to build up the patient's resistance, improving his well-being and helping to prevent relapses, for example in migraine or asthma. In chronic disease where the main complaint is pathological, as in severe rheumatoid arthritis, we can prescribe a constitutional remedy by seeking out the whole personality of the patient, with his fears and sensitivities, and his emotional reactions to people and environment, as well as the pathological symptoms. This does not alter the basic personality of the patient but improves his health, and often also his pain, stiffness and mobility as well.

Foubister (*British Homoeopathic Journal*, 1963) commented:

'Although certain polychrest remedies do seem to produce good results when given to related constitutional types, many patients cannot be so classified. There are only a few of these remedies, and there is a danger that the inexperienced may attempt to fit patients into types as part of their search for a remedy covering the totality of symptoms. If the totality of symptoms are covered, the correct prescription can almost always be found. If it should happen that the patient can be classified as belonging to a known group or type at the time of prescription, this could be an additional indication, but it is not a necessity.'

There is always the risk that we progressively restrict our prescribing to the well known polychrests, and fail to use the many other remedies with clear drug pictures, but which are not associated with types.

The constitutional picture of a patient may well be the normal personality of the patient, but often in illness this may change and a different picture presents. The symptoms and reactions at the time of prescribing are the ones to use in selecting the remedy, particularly if they differ from the patient's usual behaviour.

In conventional medicine we are aware that people belong to particular groups – blood groups, tissue groups, somatotypes. Certain groups may be more prone to certain illnesses, or have particular sensitivities. There is no reason why certain groups of patients should not respond better to particular homoeopathic remedies.

Our aim in any case is the same – to attempt to improve health and provide a sense of wellbeing. To effect real cure in chronic illness, these broad deep-acting remedies are essential – local prescribing will usually only palliate.

CHRONIC ILLNESS

Diseases can be broadly classified as acute or chronic. A true acute disease is not deep-seated and can be completely cured by a well-selected homoeopathic remedy, or else will recover on its own due to the patient's natural recuperative powers. Some acute diseases seem to recur, and this may be due to the fact that they are not acute diseases as such, but acute exacerbations of an underlying chronic disease. These will not clear up with one remedy, but may need several remedies in succession, and often a fundamental remedy to follow an acute one.

Chronic diseases are a result of many factors in the patient's history, including inherited predisposition, as well as the influence of disease in parents or grandparents. We now know the importance of genetic inheritance, and the effect on a child of illness during pregnancy. Hahnemann maintained that much chronic illness was due to suppression of disease, particularly skin disease or other superficial conditions which are not truly cured by local applications and drugs, but merely suppressed, leading to more deep-seated illness. Many homoeopaths believe that suppressing eczema with steroids may cause asthma to develop, i.e. a more superficial illness is replaced by a deeper one, and that cure can occur only if diseases exteriorise. That is, the patient feels better when a discharge or perspiration occurs – indeed, in the eczema/asthma syndrome the homoeopathic remedy, if correct, should first help the asthma, even if the eczema initially becomes worse. Further treatment will then cure the skin manifestations. (This is referred to in Chapter 7 as 'Directions of cure'.)

This concept of chronic disease resulting from suppression, particularly of skin ailments, Hahnemann called a miasm. Is it not possible that over the years, and even in the present day, we may be contributing to a legacy of chronic disease as a result of some forms of treatment? Certainly, we now see a great deal more chronic illness, arterial and heart disease, arthritis, cancer and psychiatric illness. This may in part be due to our ability to treat acute diseases, and the fact that people live longer, but are we also contributing to this through pollution of food and atmosphere, and even perhaps by treatment? It is a frightening thought.

It was also believed that chronic illness derived mainly from the two venereal diseases, syphilis and gonorrhoea, which were rife in the last century, and which are by no means controlled even with modern therapy. They have also left a legacy of chronic disease affecting not only the genito-urinary system but also joints, arteries, the neurological system and psychiatric illness. They may also have left hereditary traits, causing a wide range of pathological conditions not clearly related to them.

We are now aware that other infections such as diphtheria, measles, scarlet fever, tuberculosis, typhoid fever, malaria, abortus fever and amoebiasis, as well as vaccination, can lead to chronic ill health.

This concept of causal factors in chronic disease is of particular value to the homoeopathic doctor. He has in his materia medica remedies specially related to these conditions, which can often assist in helping to cure the patient of his chronic illness.

'Nosodes' are remedies prepared from disease tissue or from cultures of specific organisms, by the process of attenuation and subdivision described in Chapter 6, thus neutralising their toxicity but retaining their ability to antidote and stimulate restorative activity in the tissues of the body.

The treatment of allergies in orthodox medicine is akin to this. Homoeopathic preparations of allergens are available for this purpose and are proving effective.

This description of case-taking may seem a formidable task to the person new to homoeopathy. The whole picture may require to be built up over a number of interviews, and the general practitioner's knowledge of the family and the environment will greatly reduce the time spent on actual case-taking. Each doctor will modify his case-taking according to circumstances and as a result of experience, and indeed will evolve his own method. In chronic disease, not easily amenable to other forms of treatment, careful selection of the correct remedy will prove to be justified by the results.

REFERENCES

The Patient not the Cure, Margery G. Blackie
Homoeopathic Drug Pictures, Margaret L. Tyler
Classical Homoeopathy, Margery G. Blackie
The Handbook of Homoeopathy, Gerhard Koehler

TABLE 5.1   ACUTE CASE-TAKING SUMMARY

The Complaint
Pain, cough, sickness, diarrhoea.
Find out the modalities – what makes it worse or better – movement, pressure, heat, cold, etc.
The character of the cough; the colour and consistency of the sputum, the vomit or the stool.

Appearance
Flush, pallor, sweat, delirium.
Rashes.
Appearance of the tongue.
Thirst or absence of thirst.
Fever – its incidence and time aggravation.

Temperament
Drowsy, restless, fearful, irritable, desiring attention or to be left alone.
Changes from the normal.
Clinical examination.

TABLE 5.2   CHRONIC CASE-TAKING SUMMARY

The Complaint and Present History
Details of particular symptoms, modalities and onset, especially where these are strange, unusual or peculiar in some way.

Past History
With particular emphasis on infectious disease, injury, vaccination or failure to recover completely.

Family History
Incidence of tuberculosis, cancer, arterial disease, allergy.

Social History
Environment, housing, marital relations, smoking, alcohol.

Physical Examination
Appearance, colouring, manner of patient.
Detailed examination of systems, diagnosis where possible and relevant investigations required.

HOMOEOPATHIC HISTORY

General Symptoms
Reactions to heat, cold, damp, frost, thunder, sea.
Perspiration: parts, character.
Time aggravations.
Position aggravations.

Foods
Appetite: improvement or aggravation from eating.
Strong desires or aversions, and foods which disagree: sweet, salt, fat, savouries, spices, eggs, fish, sugar, milk, vinegar.
Thirst: hot, cold, large, small.

Sleep
Position in, dreams, better or worse from.

Menstrual Effects
General upset or improvement before, during or after periods.
Particular symptoms of discharge, irritation, etc.

Mental Symptoms
These are among the most important in the selection of a remedy.

Will

Placid	Weepy (relieved or	Depressed
Worried	aggravated by	Guilty
Irritable	sympathy)	Jealous
Anticipatory	Sociable	Loquacious
Resentful	Withdrawn or reticent	Tidiness
Obstinate	Temper	Indifference
Rude	Sensitive to noise	Suspicion
		Sadness

Fears

Dark	Open Spaces	Failure
Alone	Heights	Crowds
Thunder	Death	Future
Enclosed spaces	Illness	

Ailments from

Anger	Sexual excesses	Reproach or
Bad news	Grief	resentment
Love	Joy	Mental exertion

Understanding

Delusions	Difficult comprehension	Loss of sense of
Hallucinations	Mental disability	proportion

Memory

Absent-minded	Errors in answers	Mistakes in speech or writing

Particular Symptoms
Related to parts or organs. These will have been covered to some extent in the present history. The importance of modalities should be stressed.

Head	Face	Rectum
Eyes	Mouth	Genito-urinary
Ear	Respiratory	Back
Nose	Stomach	Extremities
Throat	Abdomen	Skin

CASE HISTORIES

In order to illustrate the case-taking procedure I have included a few case histories, not because they are particularly dramatic, although all but two of the patients were helped considerably. They describe the steps in taking the case and the sort of assessment one can make, especially from general and mental symptoms.

It is interesting that the three patients with dermatitis each required a different remedy, depending on their general and mental symptoms.

Case-taking Signs

In the case-histories the signs > and < are used. They indicate the modalities of a symptom, being used in the homoeopathic literature to signify:

better from or relieved by, >
worse from or aggravated by, <

For example: pain relieved by (>) heat, pressure, motion; or pain worse (<) from cold, pressure, rest.

On making a prescription, the name of the remedy is followed by the required potency (see Chapter 6) and then by the number of doses; e.g. Lycopodium 30c/3 or Pulsatilla 10M/3.

Mrs C., aged 45

Complaint

Pain and tightness in her chest for 2 years.
Nervous symptoms.

Present History

Five years ago had her left breast removed and radiotherapy to follow, causing some fibrosis of her lungs. She was complaining of pain and tightness in her chest for 2 years, worse on walking uphill or on stairs. Also breathless with a sensation of fluttering. Nervous symptoms. Cannot concentrate, upset by the death of her mother two years ago from cancer – she was very attached to her. Had tranquillisers and anti-depressants until 6 months ago. Spells when she cannot cope, is tired, irritable and weeps on talking. She is restless, fidgety and depressed in the mornings. Does not want company, and keeps her feelings to herself. Easily startled by noise. Unhappy in her present house.

Past History
Appendix removed.

Family History
Husband has bronchitis – tends to be depressed.
No family.
Father alive – stays with another daughter.
Mother died of cancer 2 years ago.

Social History
Non-smoker. Lives in a council house.

Homoeopathic History
Generals
< from extremes of heat or cold.
Sleep: poor.
Appetite: fair.
   Desires: plain food, eggs, cheese. Not thirsty.
   Aversion to: pickles, fat.
Bowels regular: some spasms of rectal pain and piles.
Urinary frequency.
Menses: had X-ray menopause at 40.
Has lost her libido and this worries her for her husband's sake.

Mentals
The mental symptoms have been described in the history as they are
   predominant.
She was a dark-haired woman, of medium build. The left breast scar was
   satisfactory and the right breast normal.

With the history of emotional upset over her mother's death, dislike of
company and sympathy, and her tendency to weep and to keep her
feelings in, the remedy Natrum Mur. was indicated.

   There were no marked food cravings or weather reactions.

   This remedy relieved her chest pain and fluttering and restored her
emotional reactions to normal within four weeks. It was only repeated at
two months and five months intervals.

Mr R. M., aged 26

Diagnosis
Ulcerative colitis.

Present History
Ulcerative colitis for several years. 5 years ago had barium enema and sigmoidoscopy and attends hospital regularly. Spells of diarrhoea and constipation – now two stools daily with some blood and mucus. No severe pain, weight steady. Anxious to stop drugs. Has had prednisolone enemas and then sulphasalazine 8 daily, now down to 4 daily. Codeine Phos. if loose stools.

Past History
Assaulted by a man when 7 years old.
Serious car accident 2 years ago.

Family History
Wife alive and well; one boy.
Mother alive and well.
Father had stomach ulcers.

Social History
Non-smoker.
Own business as electrician. Was rather unhappy during his college apprenticeship.
A slim man with blue eyes, good colour, scar on his face from car accident.
Tongue clean, no abdominal tenderness.

Homoeopathic History
Generals
Likes heat but worse in a stuffy atmosphere.
Sweaty feet, rather warm.
Appetite: good – on high protein, low roughage diet.
  Desires: sweet, meat, takes vegetables liquidised, cold milk.
  Aversion: curries, much fat.
Sleep: normal.

Mentals
Shy man, anxious, gets keyed-up on anticipation.
Living in a caravan and altering his house – a bit worried about this.

Occasional temper – not very irritable.
Not weepy or startled. Fairly tidy.
Fear of shut-in places, heights.
If he has something on his mind he likes to get it done.

An anxious man with colitis, easily keyed up in anticipation; liking for sweet food.
    Lycopodium 30c/3 prescribed.

He continued to have some urging to stool and blood and mucus, and Mercurius Cor. 6x was given twice daily for 2 months, and a further dose of Lycopodium 30c in 4 months' time. In 6 months he was much improved with normal stools, no blood or mucus, and only occasional sulpha-salazine. On follow-up a year later he had stopped all medication and was very well.

Mrs A., aged 40

Condition
Migraine for 4 years.

Present History
Migraine headaches began when under stress.
She worked for her husband in business, nursed her mother-in-law who
    died, and her own mother who was ill.
Has moved house in the last 2 weeks.
The headaches have been worse in the last 18 months, increasing in
    frequency – now nearly every week and lasting 3–5 days.
Occasionally spots before her eyes. Pain settles above the left eye; she has
    to lie down, and vomits.
She had been investigated: X-ray skull, blood, etc. Only slight anaemia.
She had been on several conventional migraine drugs, which helped her
    attacks to some extent but tended to upset her. Sometimes she has
    required an injection.

Past History
Squint in left eye as a child.
Appendix operation at 36 years.
No known allergies.

Family History
Husband alive and well.
Two daughters both well.
Mother alive and well. 72 years.
Father died aged 61 – myocardial infarction.
Twin brother died of leukaemia.
No family history of migraine.

Social History
Lives at home with husband and two daughters.
Not working now.
Non-smoker.

Homoeopathic History
Generals
Weather no effect.
Damp no effect.
< stuffy room or extreme heat.
Likes fresh air.
Dislikes tight things around her neck.
No perspiration.
Sleep: normally good. For a time waking 5.a.m. with palpitations.
Appetite: good. Has tried stopping cheese and chocolate for her migraine.
    Desires: sweet, tasty.
    Aversion: fat.
    Not thirsty. Likes hot drinks.
Other systems – NAD.
Menses: regular, occasional backache the first day.

Mentals
Generally placid – used to be upset in anticipation, but less so now.
Shy person. Although she is quite sociable, does not go out a lot.
Emotional, weeps easily. Not sure if she likes sympathy.
Shares her worries.
Very tidy.
Fear of heights, and of her headaches.

Pulsatilla was indicated from her dislike of heat and hot places, a liking for sweet food and her shy emotional personality.

   This patient received Pulsatilla 30c/3 with Bryonia to use as an acute headache remedy, which helped. She steadily improved, resumed a full-time job and had no further severe headache. Minor headaches gradually reduced, and she had only one repeat of Pulsatilla six months after her first dose and has remained well.

Mrs M., aged 56

Complaint
Huskiness of throat, headache, pressure in sinuses, and post-nasal drip.

Present History
She is a trained singer and her voice keeps going hoarse. Also nervous and
weepy since her husband died 5 years ago, weeps every day and feels a
lump in her throat.
She has had antibiotics and a nasal decongestant with little relief.

Past History
From 13–16 years she had diabetes which cleared up with diet.
Disc trouble helped by manipulation.
D and C – fibroids present.

Family History
Married twice. Divorced first husband. Second husband died with
disseminated lupus erythematosus and heart attack.
One daughter alive and well – married.

Social History
Lives alone. Non-smoker.
Sings with choir and opera chorus.
A thin woman with injected throat. Normal blood pressure.

Homoeopathic History
Generals
< excessive heat, but also < cold.
Some flushes.
Appetite: spells of nervous eating.
  Desires: chocolate, savouries.
   Aversion: pickles, fat, eggs. Thirsty at times.
Some heartburn, bowels regular.
Bladder: up twice at night.
Menses: stopped after husband's death 5 years ago.
Sleep: good.

41

Mentals
Usually happy but weepy now most days.
Anxious, worries, talks quite a lot.
Good mixer – rather sentimental but says she doesn't expect sympathy.
Affectionate.
Fairly tidy. Sensitive to smells and smoke.
Fear of dying. Noises upset her.

Here we have a lady who has a lot of catarrh and sinus trouble, with loss of voice. She is nervous and emotional since the death of her husband, lonely, affectionate and weeps frequently. No very marked food cravings. Although chilly she dislikes much heat.

Pulsatilla 10M/3 prescribed.

Six weeks later she reports feeling much better in every way. Her breathing is easier, sputum comes up more easily, her headaches are improved, she is singing clearly and, although still a bit emotional, is feeling mentally much improved.

Mrs. S., aged 44

Diagnosis
Ulcerative colitis.

Present History
History of ulcerative colitis for 3 years. Had been in hospital 1½ years ago, when the condition was diagnosed. She was on sulphasalazine and prednisolone enemas, improved for 6 months and then relapsed, with loss of weight and depression. 3 months ago she had more bleeding and last month was on prednisolone 10mg daily and steroid enemas. She was anxious to try homoeopathy to see if she could reduce her medication.

Past History
Tendency to diarrhoea if upset.
6 years ago a spell of weakness of her right arm and leg thought to be possible multiple sclerosis. Steroids given and improved. Still a little weakness.

Family History
Husband had tuberculosis – a lot of worry over him.

Homoeopathic History
Generals
Chilly person but with hot hands and feet in bed.
Sweat of feet and hands.
Appetite
  Desires: savouries, eggs.
  Aversion: fat, salt, sauces.
Menses: regular.

Mentals
Sociable person, weepy, sympathetic, better from consolation.
Untidy, startled easily, worries, gets keyed up.
Fears thunder.
Nightmares of death.

A sensitive outgoing person, untidy, emotional, better from consolation with fear of thunder and dreams. Chilly, liking for savouries, thirsty for cold drink. History of colitis with bleeding.

This picture suggested Phosphorus, which was prescribed in 30c potency, 3 doses.

Steady improvement after this, gradual reduction of cortisone which was stopped in 3 months.

Phosphorus repeated after 8 months. Two years later slight recurrence after an antibiotic for a throat infection. Gaertner 30c/3 given, the related bowel nosode (see Chapter 21.)

Reports 3 years later – no further relapse, very well, no medication.

Mr R., aged 42

Complaint
This man, who was an engineer and worked with synthetic oils, came
  complaining of a rash on his hands and feet for 4 months following a
  domestic upset. He had also been off work for 9 months.
His palms and soles were covered with small itchy blisters which burst and
  wept moisture.
He had been using steroid creams and taking diazepam.

Past History
Nil.

Family History
Wife under psychiatric care – she had been running up debts.
One daughter.

Social History
Smokes 40 per day. Drinks some beer. Plays tennis and badminton.

Homoeopathic History
Generals
> heat. < cold.
Appetite: good.
   Desires: pickles, salt, sweet, some fat, cheese, eggs.
Sleep: good.
Other systems: nil.

Mentals
Worries.
Irritable – slow to reach a temper.
A bit self-conscious, upset in anticipation.
Tidy and exact.
Likes to be busy, frustrated at being off work.
Can be a bit emotional.
A tall grey-haired man.

A chilly patient, with liking for tasty, salty foods, tidy in his habits, but
irritable and frustrated.
   Nux Vomica 30c was prescribed.
   Within 10 days his feet were improved and his palms less moist and not
so itchy. He was keen to get back to work.
   Within a month his hands were almost clear and he had started a clerical
job.

Mrs E., aged 60

Present History
Dry, cracked skin lesions on both hands and wrists, and spots on her back
   for several years.
Catarrh, blocked nose, loss of smell.
Nervous, excitable and weepy.
Nursed her mother-in-law for 8 years – she died last year and she misses
   her. She also misses her job as a theatre nurse.

Past History
Catarrh and wheezing after being in the USA.

Family History
Husband alive and well.
Two children both married – high blood pressure during second pregnancy.
Mother had thyroid operation – died of pneumonia at 81.
Father died of a stroke at 79.

Social History
Lives with her husband.
Smokes 20 per day.

Homoeopathic History
Generals
< heat. > cold.
Appetite: good.
  Desires: savouries, salt.
  Aversion: sweet, pickles, fat.
Thirst for water and coffee.
Bowels regular.
Catarrh and wheezing.
Back trouble with a disc – now improved.
Menses: stopped at 52.
Sleep: wakes early – difficult rising.

Mentals
Nervous, easily startled, upset in anticipation.
Weepy – upset by sympathy.
Used to like people but cannot now be bothered going to the shops.
Not irritable, but rather restless and impatient.
Average tidy. No fears.
Although she nursed her mother-in-law for years she found her very demanding, and was resentful about this, though less so now.

A fair, plump, rather overweight lady with a slight tremor. No thyroid enlargement.
  BP 220/115.
  Dry eruption on hands, wrists and back, thickened nails.

With the history of some resentment, nervousness, startled by noise, weepy but upset by sympathy, together with < heat, desire for salt and a skin eruption probably of nervous origin, Natrum Mur. 30c was prescribed.

This remedy helped her emotionally, her BP came down to 170/90 over the next few months and her hands healed completely in three months. She has received some other remedies for rheumatism and other complaints, but her hands remained healed.

Peter, aged 16

Complaint
This young man presented with a moist itchy eruption on his hands, of 3 years duration. Two years previously his mother had left the family and his skin became worse. He had used a steroid ointment with only temporary effect.

Past History
Leg operation.
Some history of asthma – allergy to cats, strawberries and oil.

Homoeopathic History
Generals
Prefers some heat but no marked heat, cold or weather aggravations.
Appetite: good.
  Desires: most foods, sweet, fat, milk.
Bowels normal.
Sleep good.

Mentals
A good mixer, tendency to worry, a bit emotional, fear of the dark.
Not irritable.
Rather untidy. Artistic, fond of painting.

On the basis of the skin lesion, liking for fat and sweet food, and sociable, untidy temperament, he was prescribed Sulphur 12c and then 30c.

His skin cleared up after the first prescription, and a slight relapse two months later responded to the 30c potency.

Mark, aged 3¾

A typical child seen at Outpatients is the boy with recurring coughs and colds.

He had had repeated coughs and colds since he was a baby, seven times each winter. He developed a head cold then a cough, dry and sore, then fever, and usually had to receive antibiotics so often that his doctor and his mother were concerned.

Past History
No eczema or other illness.

Family History
Nil.
A fair-haired boy, with big pupils.

Homoeopathic History
Generals
Warm person.
Appetite
  Desires: sweet, cheese, salt, sauce, butter.
Thirst for water.

Mentals
A sociable, rather wild boy with tempers.

A hot, sociable child with thirst and liking for tasty food, sweet and butter, suggested Sulphur. This was prescribed in 30c potency. Following this, his health greatly improved and his colds and coughs disappeared.

Grace, aged 7

Complaint
Bronchitis every 6 weeks for the last 9 months, the last attack being 2 weeks ago. Numerous antibiotics.

Past History
Wheeze off and on since 9 months of age.
2 years ago acute asthma – seen at Allergy Clinic and found to be sensitive to grass, pollens and house dust, but not to animals. Injections given with slight benefit.

Attacks start as a cold, then sneezing, sore throat, wheeze and then cough with green sputum. No change at the sea.

Family History
Mother and father well.
Grandfather had asthma.
A fair, slim girl with long eyelashes and dark blue eyes.
Small tonsils, no glands. Chest clear on examination.

Homoeopathic History
Generals
Upset by heat; sweat of neck and feet.
Appetite
   Desires: onions, cheese, eggs. Quite thirsty for cold milk or water.

Mentals
Well-behaved girl, shy but makes friends.
Affectionate. Weepy when ill.
A bit stubborn, not anxious.

The picture presenting here is like Phosphorus or Pulsatilla, but in view of the fact that she was upset by heat and rather weepy, Pulsatilla 30c was given. Six weeks later mother reports that she coughed up a lot of yellow catarrh after the remedy and has then been very well. She is eating well and has had no further wheeze.

Apart from obviously incurable conditions, where the most one can expect is palliation and some relief of symptoms, there are some patients who seem to fail to respond to any form of treatment, a large group being the neurotic patients whose symptoms constantly change. There are also some patients who fail to improve with homoeopathic remedies, in spite of reasonably clear prescribing symptoms. Some may genuinely fail to react to homoeopathy. In some the doctor's failure to select the correct remedy or potency, or to extract the really relevant symptoms, may lead to disappointing results. The art of questioning and weighing up the relevance of symptoms is a very skilled one. Some physicians seem to have an intuitive gift for this.

   Below are two case histories where seemingly indicated remedies failed to act. This experience should not make the doctor give up. He should be spurred on to read more widely, to re-study the case, and even take it afresh.

Miss D., aged 43

Complaint
Diarrhoea in spells of two or three days every 3 weeks since the age of 16 years.

Present History
Periodic bouts of colicky pain followed by loose stools and burning yellow mucus lasting a few days every 2–3 weeks. Also epigastric pain with heartburn and acid risings, usually relieved by eating and worse when empty, better from warm drinks. Worse before her menses. Sinusitis and occasional migraine. Barium meal 10 years ago showed some duodenal irritation, but barium enema was negative. Treated with propantheline bromide, antacids, chlordiazepoxide. Tends to be travel sick.

Past History
Pulmonary tuberculosis and cavity 23 years ago, with phrenic crush and chemotherapy.
A laparotomy 18 years ago – appendix removed but no evidence of abdominal tuberculosis.

Family History
Mother arthritic, 83.
Father 92, in psychogeriatric hospital.
Two brothers died, one of tuberculosis.

Social History
Lives with her parents.
Works as a nursing sister.
Non-smoker.

Homoeopathic History
Generals
Better from heat, used to feel cold, hands and feet cold.
Stomach: poor appetite. Desires tasty food but upset by fried food, rich, sweet, fruit.
Sleep: good. Vivid dreams.
Nose: sinusitis, green catarrh.
Menses: regular but scanty, dysmenorrhoea quite bad before and during first 2 days of period.

Mentals
Sociable. Better from company, likes affection.
A bit irritable.
Not very worried or anxious.
Sensitive but does not actually weep much.
No fears.
Rather tidy. Fond of music.
She does not admit to any particular stress, apart from those in her work, and her old father. She has had no unhappy love affair and does not appear very anxious.

A barium enema shows a rather smooth descending colon with lack of haustral markings. No evidence of neoplasm. Barium meal and follow through showed a partial volvulus of the stomach but no other abnormality in duodenum or small bowel.

Over the past 15 months this lady has attended regularly at monthly intervals and received a number of remedies. At times she seemed a little better. She now looks well with no loss of weight, but still has epigastric pain and bouts of colic with burning yellow stools for 2–3 days every 3 weeks.

Remedies Given
Tuberculinum Bov., Graphites, Gaertner, Phosphorus, Sulphur, Nux Vom., Aloes in 30c potencies, and also low potencies of Podophyllum, Mercurius Cor. and Colocynth for colic.
She has also had bran, and a spell off milk and wheat.

Charles, aged 8

Complaint
Psoriasis since the age of 3 years.

Present History
Psoriasis began in the scrotal region and spread to cover large areas of the body, arms, legs, scalp and above the ears. Large scaly plaques, itchy and dry; scalp has a thick scale. He has been in hospital and had extensive local applications, mainly of steroid ointments which help temporarily. It usually improves at the sea and in the sun. Was aggravated after chickenpox.

Past History
Measles, chickenpox, mumps. Inoculations with triple vaccine and
    polio – no upset.
Pneumonia at 2 years.
Tonsils removed at 6 years.

Family History
Mother: has migraine.
Father: well.
Two brothers and one sister well.
Two of his uncles had psoriasis.

Social History
Family middle class, no financial problems. Father seems rather over-
    powering and intense.
A dark, slim boy, with blocked nose and warts on his hands.

Homoeopathic History
Generals
Warm child. Sweat of head and feet.
Appetite: good – eats a lot but remains thin.
    Desires: sweet, tasty foods, sauce, eggs, milk, salt.
    Aversion: fat.
Bowels regular.

Mentals
Sociable, bright boy; likes older people.
Not very demonstrative; some tempers; easily bored.
At one time destructive and talkative at school.
No fears, not very tidy, not weepy.
Likes change and new things.

Remedies Given
Tuberculinum 30c caused slight improvement and his warts rapidly
disappeared.
    His skin seemed to improve quite a lot, especially his legs, after Sulphur
and Phosphorus. Marked improvement after Morgan Co. 30c.
    His nose remained very blocked, and Bacillinum and Thuja were given
with no effect. The scalp remained bad. Sulphur and then Morgan Co. and
Graphites were repeated, all in 30c potency, single doses at monthly

intervals. The skin then began to get steadily worse and he had a further spell in hospital.

He became depressed, difficult at school, restless and rebellious. Medorrhinum, Sulphur and Staphysagria were tried. He then went to Israel to a special clinic with bathing in the Dead Sea, and rubbing the scalp with salt, and this improved him a bit; on returning, in view of the improvement with salt, Natrum Mur. was given. He is happier, but the skin remains a problem.

Skin conditions which are better at the sea often respond well to Medorrhinum, but this remedy did not help. Perhaps the remedies were changed too often, even though 4–6 weeks elapsed between each. Perhaps the potencies were wrong.

One has seen cases of psoriasis which are markedly improved by homoeopathy, and some actually cured. In other patients, seemingly indicated remedies fail to act at all. A puzzling illness!

Chapter 6

The Preparation of Homoeopathic Remedies

Homoeopathic remedies can be prepared from any substance which has either a toxic effect on the body or which exerts a chemical change on it. Remedies are prepared from plant tinctures, salts, metals, snake and spider venoms and even synthetic drugs, as well as diseased tissue (nosodes).

The technique used by the homoeopathic pharmacist is laid down with great accuracy in Hahnemann's *Materia Medica Pura*, as well as in his *Chronic Diseases*.

The standard pharmaceutical texts are: *The American Homoeopathic Pharmacopoeia* 1928, *The British Pharmacopoeia* 1882, and J. H. Clarke's *Dictionary of Materia Medica*.

In the case of insoluble substances, one part of the mother substance and nine or ninety-nine parts of an inert medium, namely coarse lactose, are triturated (ground) with mortar and pestle, usually in three separate quantities. One part of this is again triturated with nine or ninety-nine parts lactose. After three stages of trituration this material can be suspended in a fluid medium, and thereafter the technique is the same as that described below for tinctures.

Homoeopathic remedies can be used in mother tincture, diluted for either local or oral medication, or they can be prepared by the technique of serial dilution and 'succussion', or mechanical shock. These solutions are known as 'potencies', in view of the apparent increase in the power of their clinical effect with increasing stages of preparation.

There are two ranges of potency. The decimal scale (1 in 10) are designated 'x' or 'D' potencies, and the centesimal scale (1 in 100) are called 'c' potencies. In the United Kingdom a potency specified by number only, without a following letter, is taken to be a centesimal potency. The reader will find both usages in this book as well as in the literature generally. An additional range of very high potencies, called 'M' potencies, are diluted 1 in a 1000 parts between succussions, and are largely made in the USA.

The extracted mother tincture of the fresh growing plant is diluted in 40 per cent alcohol in the above two dilutions, one drop to nine or ninety-nine drops of diluent. The liquid is shaken ten times in a sealed vial, two-thirds filled (i.e. by the process known as succussion). Using a separate pipette and vial at each stage, one drop of this solution is again diluted and succussed. It is important to realise that the homoeopathic potency is not simply a highly diluted solution, but one made by this rigid procedure of serial dilution and succussion.

It is now thought that this technique may alter the physical state of the solution in such a way that the specificity of the original substance is maintained, even at high degrees of potentisation. It is probable, by the laws of physical chemistry, that a potency of 12c or higher will not actually contain a single molecule of the original substance; but in practice these high potencies do seem to be active.

We do not know why or how the potentising process works. There is a discussion on this subject in Chapter 8 ('Research').

Only certain stages of potency are used in clinical practice, the commonest being 1x, 3x, 6x, 12x, 6c, 12c, 30c, 200c, 1M (or 1000c), 10M, 50M and CM.

The remedies are available in tinctures, tablets or granules. Granules are prepared with 100 per cent sucrose as a base, inoculated with the required liquid potency. Tablets contain 20 per cent sucrose in lactose as a base.

Homoeopathic remedies are available in the United Kingdom on NHS prescription, but should always be obtained from a reputable manufacturing homoeopathic chemist. The manufacturer will supply details of the preparations, which can be issued to local chemists.

Chapter 7

Principles of Prescribing, and Administration of the Remedy

The Like Remedy

Two things are necessary for the successful selection of the similar remedy: a clear picture of the patient's symptoms and a comprehensive knowledge of the materia medica.

It has been stressed already that the symptoms characteristic of the patient as an individual, in his reaction to the causative factors in his illness, play the most important part in building up the symptom picture.

The modalities of the particular symptoms are essential in their evaluation. Above all, the whole patient must be assessed, including his physical features, general reactions, and emotional and temperamental attributes.

Having obtained a full picture of the patient, reference is made to the materia medica to find a remedy which has, as nearly as possible, a similar picture in its provings and toxicology. The importance of the mental and general symptoms of the patient should also rank high in the remedy picture if a correct selection is to be made.

Different prescribers have their own method of selecting a suitable remedy. With a good knowledge of materia medica it may be possible to see the indicated remedy clearly after taking the case, without the aid of books. It is wise to list the main symptoms with their modalities, and to note any strange, rare or peculiar symptoms. Then one should look at the patient as a whole, as described under 'Case-taking', noting the appearance and the general and mental symptoms.

Select from them the symptoms which cannot be omitted because they are so marked. Then take one of the repertories mentioned in Chapter 4, Kent's being the most commonly used, and see what remedies cover most of the listed symptoms. Next look again at the materia medica of these few remedies to decide on your choice. You can give points, 3, 2 or 1 to particular remedies, depending on the weight of the type in the repertory, and then add up the score, selecting the one with most points.

Mention has been made of using remedies known to have particular value in relation to organs and systems. Section II may prove helpful in this respect.

There are considerable differences of opinion among homoeopaths on whether or when to use high or low potencies. This is a matter for individual choice and experience. Good results are obtained with either method.

The Single Remedy

The concept that the remedy acts as a stimulus to the tissues of the body, and that its selection is based on the materia medica picture, supports the view that wherever possible a single homoeopathic remedy should be prescribed. Occasionally a high potency of one remedy is given, followed by a low potency of a remedy with more local tissue affinity. This is discussed more fully under 'Administration of the Remedy' (below).

The single-remedy method of prescribing is based on the views of Hahnemann and Kent (of America) and is the one mainly used in the British Isles, in the USA and in South America. In many other countries, and notably in France and Germany, a system of polypharmacy is used by many doctors. With this method, several remedies are combined in the one preparation and are prescribed mainly on pathological indications, apparently with considerable success.

The Single Dose

Again, the concept that the remedy acts as a 'trigger effect' to the body's natural reaction points to the necessity for a single dose – the minimum stimulus required. In chronic disease this is usually given as three powders 4-hourly of a high potency – 30c or 10M. The effect of this dose may last for some weeks, and even occasionally for 2–3 months. *As long as improvement is continuing no further dose should be given.* On the other hand, recent observations suggest that in some chronic illnesses, repetition of the remedy, even in the 30th potency, daily or weekly, may in fact be beneficial.

In acute illness the stimulus of this dose will be rapidly used up and a further dose will be necessary, the speed of repetition depending on the acuteness of the condition, usually at 2–hourly intervals to begin with and then 4–hourly. In a very acute state a remedy like Carbo Veg. or Arsenicum Album may be required every 5 minutes.

The Homoeopathic Aggravation

Because the remedy causes the patient to react, it may result in some initial aggravation of symptoms. A skin lesion may become more irritable, coryza or wheezing may get worse. This is not always a bad thing as it means that the patient is reacting, and after the first week in a chronic disease improvement will usually follow. This aggravation is seldom seen in acute illness, and only in some chronic cases. It is usually not very severe but may cause some concern, for example, where a child's eczema seems initially to be getting worse. An explanation to the parent or patient that this will soon subside is usually all that is required. It is important, therefore, in chronic cases not to see the patient too often, or the prescriber may be tempted to change the remedy instead of allowing the aggravation to subside and improvement to start.

Non-interference with remedy action should be stressed again, as long as improvement is occurring.

Directions of Cure
An interesting observation in medicine in general, but in homoeopathy in particular, is the fact that if a remedy is curing the patient, symptoms and signs will progress in a particular direction.

From within outwards.
From above downwards.
From more important to less important organs.
In the reverse order of their development.

The eczema/asthma syndrome is a good case in point. Asthma is the more important and inner affection, and in curing this the eczema may become worse at first – which is the correct direction of cure.

Occasionally a patient with a severe chest or gastric disorder who is improving may notice the recurrence of a skin lesion or discharging ear, apparently 'cured' many years before. Perhaps it was merely suppressed and the more serious ailment developed. Now it is recurring, and it too will eventually be cured. (See also Chapter 5.)

ADMINISTRATION OF THE REMEDY

As already stated in Chapter 6, these are available as tinctures, granules or tablets.

Tinctures
Tinctures may be applied locally as a solution, usually 10 drops to half a pint of water, e.g. Calendula lotion for wounds and cuts, Arnica lotion for bruises. A number of ointments are also available for local application. (See Chapter 9 on injuries and accidents.) Tinctures are sometimes given

orally as drops, e.g. 5 drops three times daily of Crataegus, Iberis or Convallaria in heart conditions.

Low potency solutions of 1x or 3x are available for oral use, e.g. Hydrastis, Kali Bich. or Pulsatilla for catarrhal states.

Tablets
Both high and low potencies are available as tablets. Most low potencies, such as 1x, 3x and 6x are given in this form, one tablet two or three times daily over periods of some weeks. These are often prescriptions for local tissues or organs, e.g. Sulphur for the itch of skin lesions, Carbo Sulph. for venous stasis and congestion, Hamamelis in venous thrombosis. These low potencies can also be given in acute conditions, repeated every 2 hours, and First Aid kits often contain such tablets for colds, coughs, injuries and early fevers.

Granules
Some doctors use granules, made up in small paper packets or powders. Less than a salt-spoonful is necessary for each dose, only a few granules having the desired effect when placed in the mouth or below the tongue. The exact quantity is not important but the intervals of repetition are. The same dose can be given to infants, adults or the very old. Most potencies from the lowest to the highest are available in this form. Quantity is not important because the remedy is merely acting as a stimulus to body response, and not as an ongoing pharmacological dose.

Prescription
A typical prescription on FP10 would read as follows:

    Rx   LYCOPODIUM 30c
           3 doses (granules or tablets)
           One 4-hourly
              or
    Rx   RHUS TOX. 6x tablets
           One twice daily
           Mitte 7g.

What Potency Do I Prescribe, and When?
The potency most commonly used in the United Kingdom is the 30c, for both acute and chronic illness. High potencies, 30c, 200c, 1M and 10M are used in cases of acute illness and in patients with strong mental symptoms in their case picture. They may also be used in deep-seated chronic illness.

Mention has been made of the use of tinctures and low potencies already. They are most useful as local organ or tissue remedies, although some doctors prescribe low potencies in every case. They are also of value for prolonged use when there is severe pathological change, e.g. Bryonia or Rhus Tox. 6c in chronic arthritis. These low potencies are in small but material doses.

In *acute disease* the remedy stimulus must be repeated frequently, as already stated, and a powder or tablet may be given every 2 or 4 hours, or in very acute states every 5 minutes. When prescribing in the home, this can best be done by giving one powder or tablet dry, and dissolving one in half a cup or glass of cold water. The solution is stirred and a teaspoonful given every 2–4 hours. After the remedy is finished the cup and spoon should be thoroughly washed and scalded, or put in a hot oven, before being used again. If the remedy is changed during an illness it is wise to use a fresh cup and spoon.

The reason for scalding or dry heating a cup or spoon or medicine glass is to ensure removal of potency from the surface, and was recommended as a result of laboratory experiments by the late W. E. Boyd of Glasgow. It is unlikely that a potency leached into glass would affect another person drinking from the glass. However, potency energy is so little understood that it is possible another remedy added to the same glass without adequate cleaning could become contaminated, and thus fail to act.

It should be stated again that half a salt-spoonful of granules or one tablet is adequate for each dose; repetition is what increases the effect in acute illness, not the size of each dose. A 30c or 10M potency is usually given; and the *same* dose and potency can be given to an infant, a grown man or an elderly lady. In acute situations it may be necessary to change the remedy if a response is not seen within a few hours, or certainly the following day. The correct homoeopathic remedy acts very quickly. Carbo Veg. or Arsenicum Album should show an effect within 5–10 minutes, and remedies in pneumonia or tonsillitis will help as fast as an antibiotic, if selected accurately.

In *chronic disease* a single or divided single dose should be given as already mentioned.

This should be allowed to act as long as improvement is taking place, particularly if the patient feels better in himself, even although the local symptoms have not yet cleared up entirely. If relapse occurs with the same symptoms, a repeat dose is called for, either of the same potency or the next higher potency. If there is no improvement after 2–3 weeks, or the symptom picture has changed, a different or related remedy may be required.

The Second Prescription

When a patient returns for his second visit the doctor must attempt to assess any progress. This requires experience, as well as the ability to judge critically what the patient tells you about any aggravation, initially or continuing, and any improvement. Is the improvement in a local symptom, or in his general well-being, or in his mental and emotional state? The latter are often more important than a purely local improvement in a pain or swelling, even though this may be the patient's main complaint. There are some patients who quickly say they are better, to please the doctor; others are very reluctant to admit any change, but on questioning are found to have considerable improvement in certain aspects of their health. Do not accept the first 'I am better' or 'I am no better' immediately. Go back through your list of symptoms from the first interview, with their modalities, and find out whether they are different or better, and in what way. In particular try to assess whether the patient is 'better in himself'.

The choices open to you are to leave the remedy to continue acting, and if you feel it necessary, to give placebo; to repeat the same remedy in the same potency; to change the potency; or to select a new remedy on the symptoms *now* presenting. A graphical way of assessing your last prescription and deciding on the next is given in Table 7.2.

TABLE 7.2   DEDUCTIONS FROM EFFECTS OF THE REMEDY

1. *No change*

May mean	a) remedy wrong
	b) potency wrong
	c) patient sluggish in reacting
	d) slow-acting remedy
Reassess.	e) remedy inactive

2. *Steady rapid improvement, without any aggravation*

This means   a) remedy and potency exactly correspond, or
                  b) disease not deeply rooted

No further remedy – allow action to continue.

3. *Sharp aggravation, then quick improvement;
the improvement being long lasting*

This means

    a) remedy correct
    b) reaction vigorous
    c) no tendency to structural changes
    d) good prognosis

Patients usually do best who get this homoeopathic aggravation.
If the chief complaint is worse, but energy and emotional
symptoms are improved – wait.

61

4. *An aggravation followed by return of old symptoms,*
   in reverse order of their appearing.

> This is the best we can desire – **and the doctor must not interfere.**
> These old symptoms usually disappear in a short time – if some of
> them persist, they rank high in the next prescription.

5. *Long aggravation with slow improvement*

> Means case with much pathological change and low vitality.

long
aggravation

slow
improvement

> Do not repeat too soon – wait till patient has sufficient strength to
> react to another dose.

6. *Long aggravation with slow decline of patient.*

> Means case with irreversible pathology, or potency too high for
> feeble reaction of patient.

long
aggravation

slow decline

> The remedy may still alleviate symptoms.

PRECAUTIONS WHEN USING HOMOEOPATHIC REMEDIES

A great many rigid rules were laid down in the past, regarding what patients should or should not do when taking remedies. Some of these perhaps go to unnecessary extremes, but certain suggestions may be helpful.

The remedy should be taken when the mouth is clean and not contaminated by food, drink, tobacco, peppermint or strong toothpaste.

As far as possible, other drugs should not be taken along with homoeopathic remedies, although in certain situations this is unavoidable. Large amounts of coffee and tea can be classed as drugs.

Remedies should not be exposed to strong sunlight and should be kept away from strong odours, e.g. camphor, which is included in many proprietary inhalants or 'rubs', mothballs, menthol, and eucalyptus. Patients should preferably avoid these things while taking their remedy, as they may interfere with its action.

Chapter 8

Research

SCIENTIFIC EVIDENCE OF HOMOEOPATHIC PRINCIPLES

There are two fundamental principles underlying the practice of homoeopathic medicine. Both have already been mentioned:

1) The Simile Principle
2) The Activity of Potentised Preparations

The idea and use of a simile principle did not originate with Hahnemann or with the introduction of clinical homoeopathy. It can be traced back through history, even to the time of Hippocrates. A review of this can be found in Linn J. Boyd's book *The Simile in Medicine.*

Coming nearer to the present day, I have already mentioned that we may well be using the homoeopathic principle in conventional medicine without being aware of it, whenever we treat a patient with something which is also known to cause similar symptoms. The use of an identical substance, in potency, to that which caused the symptoms, may more accurately be described as 'isopathy'; for example, a potency of penicillin to clear up the allergic rash caused by penicillin. This has been demonstrated in a wide range of allergic conditions, but is still a kind of simile action. The use of vaccines and desensitising agents also comes within this definition.

Homoeopathic doctors have been potentising tissue and discharges from patients with measles, tuberculosis, diphtheria and septic lesions for many years, and using these remedies to treat patients. It is usually done when the patient 'has never felt well since' an illness, or has residual damage from it, rather than as a direct treatment in the acute situation.

Immunological research has developed widely in the last few years, demonstrating the importance of the reaction of the patient's own cells and antibodies to outside stimuli, or even to those within himself, varying from individual to individual. The importance of the patient's reaction, and the variations of response in individuals, has always been a fundamental of the homoeopathic approach to a clinical problem.

PROVINGS

Mention has been made of the technique of 'proving' remedies by giving repeated doses to healthy volunteers, and thus provoking symptoms, which go to form the 'drug pictures' of the materia medica. While this is valuable for obtaining data about new substances which could be used in treatment, the technique of 'proving' is also a form of trial, as the doses given are often in potency form as high as 30c or 200c. Controls using placebo are included, and the crossover method also is frequently used. These provings are themselves demonstrations of potency action, and have been recorded over many years in the *British Homoeopathic Journal* and in foreign journals. They are continuing with even more rigid control at the Royal London Homoeopathic Hospital. Demarque[1] has documented this work well in an article in the *British Homoeopathic Journal* (1987).

LABORATORY EVIDENCE OF ACTIVITY OF HOMOEOPATHIC POTENCIES

A very full review of research literature was carried out in 1982 by Kollerstrom[2] and in 1984 by Schofield[3] and published in the BHJ. These unfortunately concluded that only a few papers really stood up to critical analysis. However, some of the previous papers and other more recent research is worth studying.

W. E. Boyd[4] (Glasgow 1954) published a paper demonstrating the effects of 30c potencies of mercuric chloride on a starch-diastase preparation, and also experiments on frog heart preparations. This paper shows overwhelming statistical evidence of activity at 30c potency.

While it is now accepted that measurable effects can be recorded up to dilutions of 10^{-15}, this in homoeopathic terms is no more than a potency of 8c. Ian A. Boyd[5] has demonstrated the clear effects of perfusion of 10^{-19}g/ml acetylcholine on sensitised frog hearts. However, homoeopaths frequently use far greater dilutions in their potencies, with apparent clinical effects. It should be reiterated that a potency of 30c is not merely a dilution of 10^{-60}, but a preparation resulting from serial dilution in stages of $100^{-1} \times 30$, with succussion or mechanical shock between each stage. It is this serial dilution with succussion which we believe to be vital in the production of a potency, which may not act on a material level at all, but by means of some energy source preserved in the solvent. Theories about this have been discussed by Barnard[6] and Stephenson (1967). These theories have been further explored by Resch and Guttman[7] and published in a recent book, *Scientific Foundations of Homoeopathy*, now available in an

English translation. These new concepts have much wider implications in the world of physics.

E. Heintz[8,9] (1958, 1964, 1970, 1973) demonstrated effects of potencies up to 18x on the behaviour of fish under controlled conditions.

Boiron and Zervudacki[10] (1963, 1967) studied the effects of potencies of disodium hydrogen arsenate (3x to 19x) on the respiration of wheat coleoptiles.

Netien, Boiron et al.[11] (1966) carried out a series of experiments to demonstrate the effect of potencies of copper sulphate (15c) on plants poisoned by copper sulphate.

Cier et al.[12,13] (1967) published papers demonstrating the influence of preliminary treatment with Alloxan 9c on the diabetogenic action of alloxan on mice, and also its use after injections of alloxan. This is an interesting paper.

Boiron[14] (1973) describes the action of dilutions of 5c, 7c and 15c of copper sulphate on the respiration of *Salvinia natans*.

Fisher[15] (1982) demonstrated increased excretion of lead in lead intoxication in rats using Plumbum Metallicum in potency, and compared this with the action of penicillamine.

Keysell[16] (1984) in a simple experiment was able to demonstrate that Hypericum had an analgesic effect in mice, and that it may produce its effect in male mice by acting on the opiate receptors or causing release of endorphins and/or enkephalins.

Devenas, Poitevin and Benveniste[17] (1987) showed the paradoxical behaviour of a toxic substance when used in microdoses. Using a novel animal model based on mouse peritoneal macrophages, a highly significant increase in macrophage activity compared to control was demonstrated by a sophisticated measure of macrophage function. The animals were treated orally with Silica in dilutions equivalent to 10^{-11} and 10^{-19}. Normally Silica is toxic to macrophages.

This paper was reviewed in the BHJ in July 1987.[18] This research is an extension of similar work by Moss, Roberts and Simpson at Glasgow University in 1982, when they studied the movement of guinea-pig peritoneal macrophages and human leucocytes in inflammatory conditions when potencies of Silica 8x and some others were added to the solution.

Devenas, Poitevin and Benveniste[19] (1988) in a recent important international research experiment published in *Nature*, have demonstrated that dilutions of anti IgE subjected to vigorous shaking cause degranulation of human basophils. These dilutions were in the range up to 1×10^{120}, which is far beyond the dilution at which molecules remain in a solution. This might indicate transmission of biological information by means of the molecular organisation of water, which is a theory put forward previously by homoeopathic researchers.

Since the publication of this paper, *Nature* has sent a team of three investigators to the French laboratory to observe a series of experiments. Their report concluded that there is no substantial basis for the claims, but Benveniste argues that the investigators were unqualified to assess the results and that they carried out their observations in an unscientific way.

The matter can only be resolved by a further peer review, with adequate knowledge of the technique and an unbiased assessment. If these results are repeatable and true, they will have considerable implications for science in general and not just for homoeopathy.

Devenas et al.[20] also showed that Apis (bee venom) inhibits the degranulation of basophil cells, to which it is usually toxic, if prepared by the homoeopathic method to a dilution of 10^{-22}. See also Poitevin et al.[21] (1988).

Harisch, Kretschmer and von Kries[22] (1987) studied the release of histamine in rat peritoneal mast cells, after pretreatment with Sulphur, Silica and Calcarea Carbonica in the potencies 6x, 12x, 30x, 200x. With some potencies the release of histamine was increased and with others decreased, compared to controls.

Theories of so-called energy medicine are now being explored. Instruments are now capable of measuring the electromagnetic field of the body. A homoeopathic remedy may have a resonant frequency which can interact with a frequency produced by the body tissues, and thereby bring about a state of equilibrium where this has been disturbed during illness. It may be possible to increase the intensity of the electromagnetic field of a substance by means of potentisation. Claims are now made that selection of a homoeopathic remedy by matching the frequencies of the patient's own field and the frequencies of the remedy is possible using bio-energetic regulatory techniques (the Segmental Electrogram and the Vegatest Method).

CLINICAL RESEARCH

Can homoeopathy be proved by clinical trials? We are always accused of failing to produce double-blind statistics of clinical results, but are these anyway as reliable as some would have us believe? Are control cases really identical to those receiving medication, in terms of age, sex, build, temperament or individual sensitivity? Many drugs are tested for their short-term relief of local symptoms, without any evidence that they cure the patient.

The double-blind technique is not easily adapted to homoeopathic prescribing, for several reasons. Only rarely does a homoeopath prescribe one remedy for a specific illness, even a sore throat or pneumonia. The remedy must be selected for the individual, even though the bacteriology may be the same.

Paterson[23] (1943) demonstrated the effects of a potency of mustard gas given prophylactically, as well as after application of the liquid gas, to volunteers in a double-blind controlled trial. This work has recently been re-analysed by modern statistical methods, which confirm the original conclusion of a protective effect from homoeopathy (Owen).[24]

In trials of anti-rheumatic drugs or analgesics, the effects are assessed on the relief of symptoms over a short period, comparing this with another drug or a placebo, in a crossover trial. In a homoeopathic prescription, the relief of pain is not necessarily the criterion of successful cure. The patient's whole well-being – his emotional reactions as well as local symptoms – must be assessed in deciding the effectiveness of a remedy.

R. Gibson et al.[25,26] (1978, 1980) carried out two series of controlled trials on rheumatoid arthritis. In the first of these, 41 patients were treated with high doses of salicylate and compared with a further 54 similar patients treated with homoeopathic remedies. Both groups were compared with 100 patients who received placebos. The patients who received homoeopathy improved more than those on salicylate, but criticism of this was based on the fact that the homoeopathic group were allowed to continue their previous orthodox treatment while the salicylate group did not. Secondly, the patients in each group were seen by different doctors.

The second trial made a rigid comparison between one group of 23 patients on orthodox first-line anti-inflammatory treatment, plus homoeopathy, and a second group of 23 patients on orthodox first-line treatment plus an inert preparation. There was a significant improvement in subjective pain, articular index, stiffness and grip strength in those patients receiving homoeopathic remedies, and no significant change in the patients who received placebo. Both groups were seen by the same two physicians and the experiment was done under double-blind conditions. The numbers were admittedly small, but the trial did show significant effects.

Reilly[27,28] in a recent simple but effective trial published in *The Lancet*, set out to try to explore the hypothesis that homoeopathic potencies are placebo. He failed to find evidence in favour of this hypothesis and in fact demonstrated the superiority of homoeopathic Mixed Grass Pollens 30c over placebo in 144 subjects with active hay fever. It should be pointed out that this was not a trial to find the best method of treating hayfever, and indeed further work would be required to decide on the best potency and dosage regimen for this complaint. It was simply a conclusive demonstration that the preparation prescribed was not a placebo.

Carey[29] (1986) carried out a double-blind trial of Borax and Candida in the treatment of vaginal discharge, with good results.

Fisher[30] (1986) did an experimental double-blind trial method in homoeopathy using a limited range of remedies to treat fibrositis.

VETERINARY TRIALS

Experiments in veterinary homoeopathy show very promising results in controlled trials on animals, where placebo effect is less likely.

Day[31] (1984) describes a trial using Caulophyllum 30c on ten farrowing sows with ten controls untreated. Prior to the trial the rate of stillbirth was around 20%, but after treatment twice weekly for three weeks before farrowing the percentage fell to 10% in the treatment group, remaining at 20.8% in the untreated group. When treatment of the whole herd of 130 sows was adopted, the piglet mortality fell during the following four months to 2.6%. When Caulophyllum was stopped in the sixth month of the monitoring period, mortality rose steadily to 14.9% by the end of the eighth month. Treatment was then reinstated and in months nine and ten mortality again fell to 1.9%.

In 1987, Day[32] did a further trial in a boarding kennel for dogs, where the incidence of kennel cough was 92.5% even with conventional vaccine. By giving a homoeopathic nosode, the incidence of cough in 214 dogs dropped to 1.9%.

Research departments, particularly in France and Germany, are continuing to produce experimental evidence of potency action. What is really required in the United Kingdom is a determined effort by several laboratories with trained expert personnel and financial support to find out what happens when solutions are serially diluted and succussed, and to demonstrate clearly that activity of some kind is present in these solutions.

Clinicians using homoeopathy have no doubt whatever that their remedies have an action other than placebo effect in their patients. Somehow this must be investigated further, not just for the sake of homoeopathy, but also because the phenomenon of the potentised solution could have repercussions on many fields of medicine, physiology and physics.

REFERENCES

1. Demarque, D. The development of proving methods since Hahnemann. *Br. Hom. J.* 1987, **76**, 71–5.
2. Kollerstrom, J. Basic scientific research into the 'low dose effect'. *Br. Hom. J.* 1982, **71**, 41–7.
3. Schofield, A. M. Experimental research in homoeopathy – a critical review. *Br. Hom. J.* 1984, **73**, 161–80, 211–26.
4. Boyd, W. E. Biochemical and biological evidence of the activity of high potencies. *Br. Hom. J.* 1954, **44**, 6–44.
5. Boyd, I. A. Homoeopathy through the eyes of a physiologist. *Br. Hom. J.* 1968, **55**, 86.
6. Barnard, G. P., Stephenson J. H. Microdose paradox: a new biophysical concept. *Am. J. Inst. Hom.* 1967, **60**, 277–86.
7. Resch, G., Gutmann, V. *Scientific Foundations of Homoeopathy.* Germany. Barthel & Barthel, 1987.
8. Heintz, E. Nouvelles experiences sur le mode d'action de dilutions successives. IXe Assises Scientifiques Homoeopathiques, May 1970, 3–17.
9. Heintz, E. Measurement of the movement of fish and other animals in response to chemical stimuli. *Experimentia* 1958, **14**, 155. *Comptes Rend. Acad. Sci.* 1958, **246**, 1309; 1962, **255**, 2283; 1964, **258**, 3572. *Proc. 28th Congress for Homoeopathic Medicine*, Vienna 1973, p. 191.
10. Boiron, J. and Zervudacki, Mlle. Action of infinitesimal dilutions of sodium arsenate on the respiration of the coleoptiles of wheat. *Ann. Hom. Fr.* 1963, 738. *Rech. Exp. Mod. Hom.*, M. Plazy (ed.), 1967, p. 19.
11. Netien, G., Boiron, J. and Marin, A. Copper sulphate and plant growth. *Brit. Hom. J.* 1966, **55**, 186. *Ann. Hom. Fr.* 1966, 130. *Rech. Exp. Mod. Hom.*, M. Plazy (ed.), 1967, p. 73, Netien, G., Graviou and Marin. *Ann. Hom. Fr.* 1965, 248, 253. *Rech. Exp. Mod. Hom.*, M. Plazy (ed.), 1967, pp. 68–72, 73–8.
12. Cier, A. et al. Experimental diabetes treated with infinitesimal doses of alloxan. *Brit. Hom. J.* 1967, **56**, 51.
13. Cier, A., Boiron, J., Vigert and Braise. Sur le traitement du diabète expérimental par les dilutions infinitésimales d'alloxane. *Rech. Exp. Mod. Hom.*, M. Plazy (ed.), 1967, 80–6.
14. Boiron, J. Action de dilutions 5CH et 15CH de sulfate de cuivre sur la respiration de *Salvinia natans. Proceedings International Congress.* Vienna 1973.

15. Fisher, P. The treatment of experimental lead intoxication by penicillamine and Plumbum Metallicum. *Proc. 35 Int. Hom. Congress*, 1982, 320–2.

16. Keysell, G. R., Williamson, K. L., Rolman, B. D. An investigation into the analgesic activity of two homoeopathic preparations – Arnica and Hypericum. *Commun. Br. Hom. Res. Group*. 1984, **11**, 32–48.

17. Devenas, E., Poitevin, B., Benveniste, J. Effects on mouse peritoneal macrophages of orally administered very high dilutions of Silica. *Eur. J. Pharmac*. 1987, **135**, 313–19.

18. Fisher. P. Research Abstract – The effect of dilutions of silica on macrophages. *Brit. Hom. J*. 1987, **76**, 162–63.

19. Devenas, E. et al. Human basophil degranulation triggered by a very dilute antiserum against IgE. *Nature*, 1988, **333**, 816–18.

20. Devenas, E., Poitevin, B., Benveniste, J. Effects of Apis (bee venom) on basophil degranulation. *J. Innov. Tech. Biol. Med*. 1986, **7**, 64–8.

21. Poitevin, B. et al. In vitro immunological degranulation of human basophils is modulated by lung histamine and Apis Mellifica. *Br. J. Clin. Pharmac*. 1988, **25**, 439–44.

22. Harisch, G., Kretschmer and von Kries (1987). Contribution to the histamine release from peritoneal mast cells in male Wistar rats. *Dtsch. tierärztl. Wschr*. **94**, 515–16.

23. Paterson, J. Report on mustard gas experiments (Glasgow and London). *Br. Hom. J*. 1943. **33**, 131–43.

24. Owen, R. M. M., Ives, G. The mustard gas experiments of the British Homoeopathic Society. 1941–42. *Proc. 35 Int. Hom. Congress*.

25. Gibson, R. G., Gibson, S. L. M., MacNeill, A. D. et al. Salicylates and homoeopathy in rheumatoid arthritis; preliminary observations. *Br. J. Clin. Pharmacol*. 1978, **6**, 391–5.

26. Gibson, R. G., Gibson, S. L. M., MacNeill, A. D. et al. Homoeopathic therapy in rheumatoid arthritis. Evaluation by double-blind clinical therapeutic trial. *Br. J. Clin. Pharmacol*. 1980, **9**, 453–9.

27. Reilly, D. T., Taylor, M. A. Potent placebo or potency? A proposed study model with initial findings using homoeopathically prepared pollens in hay fever. *Br. Hom. J*. 1985, **74**, 65–75.

28. Reilly, D. T., Taylor, M. A., McSharry, C., Aitchison, T. Is homoeopathy a placebo response? Controlled trial of homoeopathic potency with pollen in hayfever as model. *Lancet*, 1986, **ii**: 881–6.

29. Carey, H. Double-blind clinical trial of Borax and Candida in the treatment of vaginal discharge. *Comm. Br. Hom. Res. Group*. 1986, **15**, 12–14.

30. Fisher, P. An experimental double-blind trial method in homoeo-pathy. Use of a limited range of remedies to treat fibrositis. *Br. Hom. J.* 1986, **75**, 142–7.
31. Day, C. E. I. Control of stillbirths in pigs using homoeopathy. *Vet. Rec.* 1984, **114**, 216.
32. Day, C. E. I. Isopathic prevention of kennel cough. Is vaccination justified? 1987. *IJHV*, **2**: No. 1: p. 45.

SECTION II

SYSTEMATIC APPROACH TO MATERIA MEDICA

In treating a patient homoeopathically we should always try to study the patient as a whole, and seek a remedy which covers as many as possible of the patient's leading symptoms. However, in our medical training we are taught to think of illnesses in relation to the systems of the body, although more than one may be involved. In this section I have selected some of the leading remedies of value in particular diseases, and set out some of the indications for them. Indeed, there are some remedies with particular affinities for certain organs, although many will appear under several systems. A fuller description of some of these appears in Section III.

Remember that diagnosis is still important, as this may help in selection of the remedy or may indicate the need for a conventional drug, a replacement therapy, or surgery.

COMMON ACUTE REMEDIES

Aconitum
Antimonium Tartaricum
Arnica
Arsenicum Album
Belladonna
Bryonia
Cantharis
Carbo Vegetabilis
Chamomilla
Colocynth

Gelsemium
Hepar Sulphuris
Ipecacuanha
Mercurius Solubilis
Nux Vomica
Phosphorus
Pulsatilla
Rhus Toxicodendron
Sulphur

POLYCHREST REMEDIES OF WIDE ACTION

These remedies will have symptoms related to many different systems. They are frequently used and should be studied in detail:

Arsenicum Album
Calcarea Carbonica
Graphites
Ignatia
Lachesis
Lycopodium
Natrum Muriaticum

Nux Vomica
Phosphorus
Pulsatilla
Sepia
Silica
Sulphur
Thuja

Chapter 9

Accident and Injury Remedies

Most of this chapter was contributed by my colleague, Dr R. A. F. Jack, a general practitioner in rural practice with a wide experience of emergencies and accidents.

ACCIDENTS AND FIRST AID

It is in the treatment of accidents, injuries and shock that homoeopathy excels all other therapies.

The homoeopathic materia medica lists many remedies suitable for treating these conditions. For simplicity, the writer has selected those medicines which he has found most useful for first aid use in general practice during the past thirty-five years. The dosages are those of his own preference, but are thought to be in accordance with current prescribing.

Aconite
Indications
All cases of mental or physical shock or fright with any of the following symptoms: tremor, palpitations, hyperventilation or gasping for breath, tight feeling in the chest, feeling cold or hot, collapse, or obvious fright or distress. Also in eye injuries.

Examples
'My grandmother has fallen down the front steps', or 'The baby has fallen from her pram.'
'My son had just been scalded/run over/bitten by a dog.'
'She has just heard that her sister has died.'
'He has just had a near miss when a lorry ran out of control.'

These are only some of the daily urgent messages a busy general practitioner receives, and in any such emergency Aconite is indicated. The doctor should give it on arrival at the scene, not only to the patient but also to all others present who are emotionally involved. While it is acting, it gives time for the doctor to assess the situation and plan treatment, including deciding what remedy should follow.

It works best in the highest potency (10M upwards) and should be repeated every 5 to 15 minutes, according to the emergency, as it is a very short-acting, though powerful medicine. Fortunately it acts very rapidly.

In summary, the more the shock or panic, the greater the need for Aconite, and the quicker it works.

Arnica
Indications
Bruises, sprains, contusions, head injuries, concussion and post-concussional headaches and myocardial infarction. Arnica is valuable for all the above conditions. It prevents and relieves muscle fatigue from over-exertion. The Swiss guides still chew Arnica leaves to prevent or remove muscle aching and soreness.

Dosage
Use in any potency which is available – 6c, 30c, 200c or 10M. Repeat every 15 minutes in acute conditions, and otherwise every 2 to 4 hours. Locally it can be applied in a cream, or as a compress, provided the skin is unbroken. For this purpose a solution is made from 2 to 3 ml of mother tincture (designated φ) in a cupful of cold water. Arnica in high potency is so effective when taken internally that local treatment is often unnecessary.

Aconite and Arnica between them probably are indicated in 80 per cent of all accidents or emergencies, and many doctors have been converted to homoeopathy following their initial experiments and successes with these two medicines.

Calendula
Indications
Cuts, lacerations, abrasions, gravel rash, burns, sore fissures and bed sores. Used as a mouth-wash it is an excellent haemostatic after dental extraction. Also valuable externally after episiotomy.

The marigold plant has an ancient reputation as a 'vulnerary' or 'wound healer'. It promotes the formation of healthy granulations.

Dosage
Use internally in potency 12c to 200c, or apply locally in aqueous solution (10 drops of tincture in half a pint of water), oil, cream or ointment.

Carbo Vegetabilis
Indications
For collapse or faint. A valuable remedy in vasovagal attacks or in more severe collapse, post-operatively or in cardiac cases, where the patient is cold, bluish, sweaty, with cold extremities, thin thready pulse and a desire for air at a window, or to be fanned.

Dosage
30c–10M potency, given frequently either in granules dry on the tongue or in water every 5–10 minutes until response, and then at longer intervals.

Hypericum
Indications
Nerve injuries – as in crushed finger tips, painful animal bites (dogs, cats and other pets, rodents, etc.), penetrating puncture wounds such as from splinters, thorns and nails. Post-operative pain. Lacerations.

St John's Wort, like marigold, is another plant quoted by Culpeper in his *Herbal*, which for centuries has been used to relieve painful injuries to soft parts richly supplied with nerve endings. In the case of a crushed finger tip, it would be indicated if the pain persisted. Arnica is given first, to stop the extravasation of blood beneath the nail.

Dosage
As for Calendula. Hypercal ointment, containing Hypericum and Calendula, is both soothing and healing.

Ledum
Indications
The chief remedy for puncture wounds, e.g. a nail into the sole of the foot. Also of value in bruising around the eye, where it seems to be even better than Arnica. The pains of Ledum are always worse from heat and better for local cold applications.

Dosage
30c–10M potency, repeated 2–4 hourly as required. In deep, potentially septic wounds, tetanus immunisation should also be given.

Rhus Toxicodendron
The poison ivy, in potency, is indicated for the effects of strains where the muscle stiffness and aching are temporarily relieved by movement, are worse at rest, and are worst after prolonged rest. The first movements to 'limber up' after a night's sleep are the most painful.

Dosage
30c–10M potency, 2-hourly.

Ruta
Rue is ideal for treating strains of ligaments around joints, when the symptoms are 'like Rhus Tox. but more so'. Particularly where periosteal attachments are involved.

Dosage
30c potency, 2–4 hourly. Both these can follow Arnica and can be used in all potencies, repeating the dose every four hours until relief.

Staphysagria
Indications
Useful in incised wounds and therefore after operation, especially in gynaecological repairs. It relieves pain and helps healing.

Dosage
30c–10M potency, repeated 2 hourly for 6 doses.

Symphytum (Comfrey or Knitbone)
Used in lowest potencies (3x to 6x), Symphytum has the reputation of accelerating the union of fractures, and is also very useful in treating contusions of the eye.

HEAD INJURIES

Where drowsiness persists despite medication with **Arnica**, give **Opium** 30c upwards, and if there is still no improvement consider the need for **Helleborus**. It is assumed that the practitioner would admit the patient to a neurosurgical unit for observation, should his condition warrant it.

For persistent post-concussional headaches, unrelieved by Arnica, use **Natrum Sulphuricum** 30c, increasing to 10M.

INSECT AND PLANT STINGS, AND INSECT BITES

Homoeopathy certainly has more to offer than the old-fashioned treatments with blue bag, vinegar or lemon juice, and offers a satisfactory alternative to the conventional treatment with topical steroids and antihistamines.

Traditionally **Ledum** (Marsh tea) is given in low potency for bee and wasp stings, when the sting or bite is relieved by cold applications. The writer prefers to give **Apis Mellifica** (potentised honey bee) to victims of bee stings, and **Vespa Vulgaris** (wasp) to those stung by wasps. In both cases, very high potencies (10M) should be used, repeated every five minutes until relief.

As a local application, a compress of Urtica Urens (see below) is very soothing, as is Hypercal ointment.

Urtica Urens
The nettle is effective used internally in potency, and externally as a compress, for nettle stings and any allergic urticarial reactions that simulate nettle stings, provided the skin is intact.

BURNS

Both Urtica and Cantharis cause and cure burning vesication of the skin, and accordingly are used in the homoeopathic treatment of burns. They are applied in the form of ointments and creams, or Urtica lotion (10 drops in one pint of boiled water).

Cantharis should also be given internally in the 30c potency every 15 minutes to 2 hours, according to the severity of the symptoms, until relief.

Cantharis
Spanish fly in 30c potency is effective in treating gnat bites, where painful blisters result which burn when touched, and where the affected skin rapidly necroses. Pyrethrum liquid is a useful deterrent against gnat bites, and should be diluted and applied to the exposed parts of the skin.

HEATSTROKE

Belladonna
This is an excellent remedy for the effects of sun exposure, and rapidly controls the fever, headache and malaise. If the headache persists, use **Glonoine**.

CHILLING

Camphor

An excellent prophylactic against the effects of being chilled, and as such is most useful for doctors who have to do night visits. A dose taken every five minutes until warmed will usually prevent a cold or diarrhoea from developing. If taken at the onset, Camphor will abort an attack of diarrhoea, if the patient feels very cold.

It is interesting to note that Camphor was one of Hahnemann's three specifics for the treatment of cholera.

Chapter 10

Headache

CAUSES AND INVESTIGATION

When faced with a patient complaining of headache, it is important to exclude causes which may require further investigation or neurosurgery.

Extracranial

Trauma.
Myalgia and cervical spondylosis.
Eye disease.
Herpes zoster.
Tic douloureux.
Cranial arteritis.
Polymyalgia rheumatica.
Migraine.

Cranial

Dental abscess.
Otitis and mastoiditis.
Sinusitis.
Disease of skull.

Intracranial

Traumatic
  Post-concussional syndrome.
  Haemorrhage – extradural, subdural.
Inflammatory
  Meningism and meningitis. Poliomyelitis. Abscess. Sinus thrombosis.
Vascular
  Subarachnoid haemorrhage.
Neoplastic
  Primary and secondary tumour.
  Pituitary tumour.

Hypertensive
Primary
   Essential hypertension.
Secondary
   Renal.
Vascular.
Endocrine.

Psychogenic
Anxiety, hysteria.

Skull X-ray, lumbar puncture, electroencephalogram, brain scan and occasionally arteriography may be required to make a diagnosis. Teeth and sinuses should be examined and eyes tested. If hypertension is found, this may need further investigation.

If there is a history of injury, even some considerable time before, we must consider using Arnica as a first prescription, before following up with further remedies. In cases of occipital blows on the head consider Natrum Sulph., which will often deal with the persistent headache.

Where the eyes seem to be the main cause of pain, consider such remedies as Ruta, Silica and Natrum Mur., after making any necessary adjustment to spectacles. These remedies all help in eye strain and weakness of eye muscles.

Sinusitis is of course a common source of head pain and one that is often difficult to cure by orthodox means. We have a wide range of remedies available here: Aconite, Belladonna, Bryonia, Spigelia, the Kali salts, Pulsatilla.

Apart from the conditions mentioned, many patients come with a history of migraine or of headache which has no identifiable cause, and which may in some cases be psychogenic.

In homoeopathic prescribing for headache, the modalities are most important in distinguishing one remedy from another.

ACUTE HEADACHE REMEDIES

Belladonna
Throbbing headache, worse on stooping, lying, jar and noise. Flushed dry face with dilated pupils and often fever, sometimes accompanied by delirium. Also after exposure to the sun.

Bryonia
Pain often right-sided but particularly worse on movement of head or eyes and better from pressure, occurring frequently in association with a respiratory infection and cough which aggravates the pain; also of value in migraine. Wants to be left alone.

China Sulphurica
Aching pain in the occiput extending over the head. Sweaty damp head. Better from cold applications, worse on turning the head or eyes and worse in the open air. Patient looks nauseated but wants to eat. Flatulence but cannot break wind (a China symptom).

Gelsemium
This is the remedy for influenzal headache, dull, aching, occurring in damp mild weather and accompanied by the usual aching in the limbs, hot and cold sensations, and chills up and down the back. Lack of thirst, even when febrile, and drowsiness add to this picture. The headache is relieved by passage of large quantities of pale urine.

Glonoine
Bursting headache, sometimes brought on by exposure to heat of the sun, with pounding in the head, such as that found in men working with nitroglycerine. Worse bending down.

Iris Versicolor
Frontal headache or feeling of constriction of head, with bilious vomiting and nausea. May come on after mental strain, on relaxing. Headache worse at *rest*, better from motion. Useful in acute migraine.

Magnesia Phosphorica
Neuralgic type of pain, especially shooting on the right side, and a deeper occipital headache spreading over the head on the left.
Pain occurs after exposure to *cold* or nervous strain and excitement. Worse from cold air, touch, 9–11 a.m. or 4–8 p.m. Better from warmth, firm pressure.

Sanguinaria
Recurring *periodic* headache, commencing in the morning and abating in the evening. A very useful migraine remedy for right temporal or frontal pain, with dizziness and sickness, better lying down and sleep. The menstrual periods are profuse and the patient feels worse before and after

them. It is also a remedy for paroxysmal cough relieved by loud eructations of wind. Rheumatic pains in the right shoulder are also helped (Rhus Tox., Ferrum Met. also).

Sanguinaria can be given to migraine patients to use in the acute phase, and it frequently cuts short the attacks or reduces their severity.

Spigelia

Shooting pain on the left side of the head extending to the face and arm, worse on motion, stooping.

CHRONIC HEADACHE REMEDIES

In patients with persistent dull headache, or recurring headache, cure will often depend on an accurate assessment of the patient's general and mental symptoms as well as the local features and modalities of the headache itself – in other words, seeking the totality of symptoms for that particular patient. The onset and possible precipitating causes and environmental and social conditions must be studied, and may indeed help in choosing the correct remedy. Opium following fright, Ignatia after grief, or Staphysagria where there is resentment or frustration.

Migraine treated between attacks in this more constitutional way will often become less frequent, and may be cured.

Argentum Nitricum

Headache resulting from excitement, mental overwork or travelling. It has a gradual onset and sudden cessation. There is tenseness, stiffness and soreness of the back of the neck, and a feeling as if the head is drawn back. The pain spreads over the head to the left temple and the scalp is tender to touch.

Worse at noon, using eyes, motion or exertion, even talking or stooping. Better from pressure and fresh air.

The typical Argentum Nit. patient is full of anticipatory fears, with churning and wind in the stomach, fear of heights and a strong liking for sugar and salt.

Calcarea Carbonica

Headaches caused by exposure to extremes of cold or heat, overeating or overdrinking.

It is often beating in character in the right temple, and associated with eructations, gastric upset or conjunctival congestion. The head is cold and damp to touch, and Calcarea patients sweat on the head and have cold clammy hands.

The headache is worse from light, stooping, walking and alcohol, better with eyes closed, lying down and sleeping. The typical Calcarea patient is stout, pale, sweaty and slow, with fears and bad dreams.

Cimicifuga (Actea Racemosa)

This remedy is apt to be neglected but it is a most useful one for headache. The pain is often occipital or pressing out or up, as if the top of the head would fly off, and extending to the eyes. There is often rheumatism in the muscles of the neck, or neuralgia of the ciliary nerves. It is mainly a female remedy with aggravation at the menstrual period, accompanied by black gloom. The patient may even think she is going insane.

Chilliness and tendency to take cold, but prefers cool and open air for the local headache. Jerking and twitching of the muscles and changeableness in both physical and mental spheres (like Pulsatilla).

Cocculus

Headache brought on by extreme exhaustion and anxiety in nursing a sick relative. Also in sickness when travelling by car or boat, with headache, dizziness and nausea. Congestion of the head, pressing or bursting with whirling and sickness. Airsickness often responds better to Borax.

This remedy also has slowing down of the faculties, great exhaustion, paralysis and numbness.

Kali Bichromicum

Headaches at the root of the nose and spreading. Of great value in sinus trouble, either with the typical sticky white or yellow catarrh or where there is pain, without discharge. The pain is worse on motion and stooping, better in the open air and eating, especially hot things. In migraine there is dimness of vision first, then a gap and then headache.

The patient dislikes the heat, and pains occur in spots; crusting of the nose and bleeding may occur. Pains of rheumatism often alternate with the catarrh. A yellowish appearance is characteristic of the remedy.

Lachesis

Few of us would like to be without this valuable snake remedy. It is particularly helpful in menopausal patients and has a characteristic aggravation on first waking – the patient sleeps into the headache.

Pulsating hammering headache with purplish appearance of the face and puffy eyes. The blueness occurs in Lachesis generally, with ecchymoses, or congested purplish throat or legs.

This remedy is often left-sided and usually better from cold. The patient is generally worse from heat and tight constricting garments..

The mentals are marked, with jealousy, suspicion and loquacity predominating, although slowness of speech and taciturnity can also occur.

Lycopodium

This remedy is often applicable to the stresses, strains and rush of modern life. The headaches are often periodic and particularly occur when the patient is empty. He has the faint 'all gone' sensation one usually associates with Sulphur, and eating helps the Lycopodium headache. It is worse from heat, warmth of the bed and lying down, and better from cold or cold air. Right-sided symptoms are common with this remedy. In spite of the relief from eating, these patients are easily filled up, distended and have much flatus. They love hot drinks and sweet food. Aggravation of symptoms at 4 p.m. or 4–8 p.m. is a useful guide.

The Lycopodium patient is anxious and worried-looking, anticipates trouble and lacks confidence, although he is often intellectual and capable when the time comes. Dread of forgetting or making mistakes. Averse to company, especially new company, and yet a dread of solitude. Fears of crowds, of the dark and of ghosts. Sensitive and emotional – he may weep when being thanked.

Natrum Muriaticum

The Natrum headache is also hammering in type and often accompanied by visual disturbances, zig-zags or even loss of vision while reading, with watering of the eyes. It is usually worse from midday to evening, and aggravated by the sun. The patient and her head are sensitive to noise, she feels the cold but is worse from much heat, and is generally worse at the sea. This latter feature ties up with the strong liking or dislike of salt. Periodicity is a feature of this remedy in regard to many symptoms, but equally to headache.

These patients often have greasy skins with a tendency to acne, and are usually worse at the menstrual period.

The mental symptoms are often difficult to extract because the patient is nervous and reticent by nature, although she may cover this up by an appearance of self-assurance. She tends to brood and harbour resentment. The headache may occur as a result of emotional breakdown after grief or a disappointed love affair. She dislikes sympathy, but at the same time craves attention if she considers it to be due to her.

It is wise not give this remedy in the acute phase of headache, but rather perhaps its acute partner Bryonia – followed up by Natrum Mur.

Nux Vomica

A most valuable remedy for the effects of over-indulgence in eating, drinking or physical exertion. The hangover headache. But also useful with the Nux personality. The pains are often neuralgic in type. Some gastric symptoms are common, and vertigo may accompany the headache. He is fond of tasty foods, spices and fat. Nux is essentially a chilly patient, sensitive to draughts and all external impressions, light, noise and colours. He is above all irritable and fastidious.

Pulsatilla

In general, Pulsatilla is worse from heat and relieved by motion. The headaches are throbbing, congestive in type, better from cold applications and slow movement, often associated with the menstrual period and relieved after it (like Lachesis). Girls with headache when about to menstruate. Sickness may accompany the headache. This remedy is valuable in periodic attacks or the old-fashioned acidosis resulting from too fat or rich food. The Pulsatilla patient likes sweet food as well as pastries, which upset, and is not thirsty even during fever. Symptoms of this remedy are often worse in the evening – the headache, the cough, the fever. There is frequently catarrh, usually yellow. Sinus conditions are helped, particularly where the pains are worse from heat. Changeableness of symptoms is characteristic – rheumatic pains, headaches, type of stool.

The mental symptoms are well known – gentle yielding disposition, easily weepy, wants attention and sympathy but is also touchy, jealous and irritable.

Sepia

The headache of Sepia is often associated with nausea, and although occurring in pregnancy morning sickness, is usually better from sleep (unlike Lachesis). It is also improved by violent exertion. Sepia is useful for the tired, jaded, irritable housewife with backache, feelings of prolapse and desire to sit down. But if she goes to a dance in the evening she comes alive, her headache gone and her sparkle returned. Characteristically these patients are sallow and thin, feel the cold but are faint in hot, stuffy atmosphere, and flush easily.

The mentals are again helpful – irritable, weepy, usually tidy but now indifferent to her house or her family.

Silica
The headache of this remedy is often occipital, extending over the head to the eyes, especially the right. The head is very sensitive to draughts and is better wrapped up tight and warm – the old gentleman who always wears a night cap. Sometimes there is loss of half the field of vision and numbness of the arm. Bursting headache with sensitivity to noise, aggravated by physical or mental exertion.

Together with these local symptoms we have the Silica generals and mentals. Chilliness, clammy sweaty feet and hands, dread of failure, lack of confidence, lack of strength – exhausted by talking and therefore dislikes people, irritable, over-conscientious and resentful, and of course the tendency to sepsis. Silica is complementary to Pulsatilla.

Sulphur
Periodic sick headaches, occurring at seven-day intervals, often preceded by flickering and zig-zags. Headaches often occur on Sundays, when the patient lies in late – it is better when he is busy and active. There is a feeling of dullness and congestion. The head is hot and burning with relief from cold applications, but otherwise the headache is better in a warm room, worse from light, stooping, jar and after eating. Redness of the face.

The Sulphur patient is usually untidy and dirty, selfish and full of theories. Some are stout, jovial and red-faced.

Many of these remedies for headaches are common polychrest remedies with a wide range of symptoms and application. They should be studied further in Section III and in other texts. Headache is a symptom appearing in many remedy pictures.

Chapter 11

Eye Remedies

This chapter was originally written by my colleague, Dr R. D. Calcott. I have tried to enlarge it from my own experience and have added some broader headings.

Kent in his *Repertory* has a section on 'Eyes' and one on 'Vision'. These are worth studying as they have headings with modalities on pain, inflammation and discharges. Most eye conditions require specialist advice and surveillance, although homoeopathy can be of great value in both acute and chronic conditions.

CATARACT

Cineraria
Mother tincture, 2–3 drops in an eye bath of boiled water once and later twice a day – continued indefinitely. Indian physicians have claimed that this remedy will slow the development of cataract and in some cases improve it, although modern eye surgery is often essential.

Calcarea Iodata 6c, **Causticum** 6c and **Phosphorus** 6c are useful remedies. Give b.d. for 14 days with a 14-day gap, and alternate the remedies.

CONJUNCTIVITIS

Apis Mellifica
Redness, stinging, burning of the eyes with oedema of lids relieved by cold.

Argentum Nitricum
Conjunctiva scarlet red, oedematous but always purulent, again better from cold.

Arsenicum Album
Burning, acrid watery discharge, better from heat.

Calcarea Carbonica
Stickiness of the lids on waking, photophobia in a cold wind.

Euphrasia
Redness is diffuse with marked photophobia – discharges are acrid and can excoriate the lateral canthi. Frequently of value in acute coryza, hayfever and measles, both in potency by mouth and also locally, 2–3 drops of mother tincture in an eye bath.

Pulsatilla
Discharges are profuse and bland – white or yellow pus. Better in the open air, worse in a warm room. Helpful in measles.

Rhus Toxicodendron
Acute inflammation with swelling of lids, stickiness and difficulty in opening the eyelids. Early orbital cellulitis. A remedy often indicated in early shingles.

CORNEAL ULCER

Hepar Sulpharis
Perhaps the most useful remedy, especially where there is sepsis – pains are sharp, needle-like, in spasms worse at night. Worse in any draught.

Mercurius Solubilis
If there is much vascularisation round the ulcer – also worse at night. Cannot bear the light of the fire or daylight. Profuse burning, excoriating lachrymation, with mucopurulent discharge.
    The usual Mercurius features of offensiveness, perspiration and dirty mouth.

Conium
Primarily for dendritic ulcers – often with enlarged lymph glands. Weakness of sight and giddiness causing the patient to stagger.

Silica
For chronic indolent ulcers with little vascularisation. Scarring and opacities of the cornea.

DETACHED RETINA

This condition essentially requires eye surgery, but some remedies may be of value in helping healing.

Arnica
As always, for injury.

Apis Mellifica
For balloon detachment.

Hypericum
For pain following retinal surgery.

DIABETIC RETINOPATHY

Adequate control of diabetes is important, using a combination of homoeopathic and conventional approaches where required.

Syzygium
This remedy has a reputation for specific effects on diabetes and can be given in mother tincture, 3 drops daily in water. Constitutional prescribing should also be used, and here **Natrum Mur., Lycopodium** or **Sulphur** may be indicated.

For retinal haemorrhage consider **Lachesis** 1M, and also **Hamamelis** in tincture or low potency.

EPIPHORA (Watering Eyes)

Use the constitutional remedy followed by **Thiosinaminum** 3c t.d.s. for two weeks. Repeat the latter in one month and assess the results after three months.

Silica
Helpful in 6c potency b.d., particularly where the tear duct is blocked, especially in young children.

Natrum Muriaticum
Has watering eyes in cold air.

EYE STRAIN

Pilocarpus Jaborandi
Where the eyes tire from the slightest use, or where muscle weakness causes squint. **Natrum Mur.** and **Ruta** are also indicated where the muscles of the eye ache.

GLAUCOMA SIMPLEX

It is essential to seek specialist advice, particularly in the acute phase of glaucoma, so that accurate pressure measurements can be made, and drops prescribed.

Gelsemium
May also be of value in maintaining normal tension. Gelsemium 6c t.d.s. for 14 days, with three doses of 30c every seven days. Repeat this four or five times per year. Also prescribe constitutionally between courses.

Ruta
In 10M potency for sudden rises in pressure.

INJURY

Aconite
For flick on the eye. 10M potency two or three doses.

Arnica
Bruising of lids and orbit. Follow this with **Ledum** 200c.

Symphytum
Pain of the bony orbit.

ACUTE IRITIS

Mercurius Solubilis, **Mercurius Corrosivus** and **Hepar Sulphuris**. These remedies cover a high percentage of cases. The Mercury salts are characterised by acute burning, lachrymation with photophobia from heat or glare, and red, swollen, excoriated lids.

Hepar Sulphuris
Profuse secretions, usually purulent with ulceration, and usually with relief from warm applications.

CHRONIC IRITIS

This may often recur in cases of rheumatism and arthritis where constitutional prescribing is required. **Syphilinum** should always be considered in chronic recurring eye ulceration or inflammation.

MACULAR LESIONS

Lycopodium
Lycopodium 10M and the constitutional remedy followed in two weeks with **Ledum** 200c.

MEIBOMIAN CYST

Thuja
30c for the average cyst.

Staphysagria
200c where there is much oedema and redness.

Baryta Carbonica
10M for smaller, harder cysts. Kent mentions several other remedies under 'Nodules' or 'Tumors of Eyelids'.

RETINAL HAEMORRHAGE

Lachesis
1M followed by **Hamamelis** 6c t.d.s. for five days. Always remember **Arnica** for bleeding.

SCLERITIS

Thuja
A very useful remedy, and often the only one required.

SEBORRHOEIC BLEPHARITIS

This redness of the eyelids is often associated with seborrhoea of the scalp, with itch and scaling. Constitutional prescribing is best, but some of the local signs are often as follows:

Argentum Nitricum
Crusting of margins of lids, with inflammation, pain and purulent discharge.

Graphites

Crusting of the lids, with honey-like exudates and cracks in medial canthi. Usually associated with more widespread skin eruptions, psoriasis or eczema, with cracks and itching around the ears as well.

Pulsatilla

Soreness and itching of the eyelids, often in patients with measles or catarrh with bland discharges, although the eyes themselves itch and burn. Especially indicated in a Pulsatilla patient.

Natrum Muriaticum

Chronic blepharitis with recurrent meibomian cysts.

Nitric Acid

This remedy is characterised by cracks, fissures and offensive discharges. Dark rings under the lids. Often purulent lesions.

Sulphur

The typical burning, hot, itchy eruption of Sulphur applies also to the eyelids, but is usually associated with more general skin eruptions, aggravated by heat and bathing.

SQUINT (Strabismus in Kent)

Gelsemium

6c t.d.s. for two weeks followed by **Gelsemium** 30c.

Cyclamen

Eye symptoms often related to migraine. Convergent squint after convulsions and in connection with menstrual irregularities.

STYES

Again, **Pulsatilla**, **Sulphur** or **Graphites** may be indicated, depending on other constitutional features or skin lesions.

VITREOUS HAEMORRHAGE

Ledum

3x tablets for 14 days, repeat in three to four weeks.

Eye symptoms and signs appear in the materia medica of many widely-acting remedies, and may be better treated as part of a whole picture of symptoms, although some local remedies are useful in acute situations or general practice prescribing.

Chapter 12

The Respiratory Tract

(Including remedies useful in infectious fevers, sore throats, coughs and colds and early pneumonias.)

This group of illnesses forms the largest seen in general practice, and nowadays is mainly treated with antibiotics and the occasional cough medicine. It should be remembered that many of these are virus diseases not affected by antibiotics – although these drugs are still important and life-saving, they should be prescribed only with careful thought and selection. In most situations the homoeopathic doctor will be able to relieve these illnesses with the indicated remedy. After commencing with the homoeopathic remedy, it may be necessary in certain patients to add an antibiotic if the response is not adequate, or the patient is very weak, or the organism is particularly virulent, or else in the case of active tuberculosis. The majority of patients, even with pneumonia, will be cured rapidly by the correct homoeopathic remedy.

In cases of asthma it may be necessary to use a bronchodilator, an inhaler or a short course of steroids, but this should always be secondary to the selection of the well-indicated remedy.

The ability of homoeopathic constitutional remedies to reduce the recurrence rate of respiratory or throat infections, or the attacks of asthma, is one of the most satisfying aspects in homoeopathic prescribing.

ACUTE COLDS AND HAYFEVER

Allium Cepa
Coryza with streaming eyes and nose, with acrid discharge from the nose and bland discharge from the eyes. There is sneezing and headache, and the patient is hot and thirsty, worse in a warm room, better in open air.

Ambrosia
Hayfever with lachrymation and intolerable itching of the eyelids. Stuffed feeling in the nose and head. Nosebleeds.

Arsenicum Album
Thin, watery nasal discharge excoriating the upper lip, but nose stuffed up. Sneezes from every change of weather. Chilly. Burning relieved by heat. Restless, anxious, fastidious.

Arsenicum Iodatum
Raw, burning, pouring nasal discharge with nasal obstruction. Sneezing which aggravates. Dislike of excessive heat, restless.

Euphrasia
In these cases the lachrymation is acrid and the nasal discharge bland. Worse from light, warmth and better in the dark. Coryza worse in the night and lying down, but cough worse by day and better lying down.

Mixed Grass and Pollen
The 30c potency can be of value as a prophylactic if started at the beginning of the pollen season. There are different suggestions for dosage. Some prescribe a weekly or fortnightly dose, others a daily dose for two weeks at the start of the season.

There is also a hayfever mixture available from homoeopathic pharmacists. This contains several remedies and is given in 6c potency daily when symptoms are troublesome.

Natrum Muriaticum
Abundant nasal discharge and lachrymation. Sneezing violent. Dry cracked lips with herpes. Severe headache worse from heat, better from cool. Again irritable, and dislikes being disturbed.

Nux Vomica
Patient is tucked up in bed with clothes all round, even over his head. Shivers if uncovered. Aching all over, sweaty. Slight sore throat, dirty brownish tongue. Desire for warm drinks. Very irritable.

Sabadilla
Persistent, violent, abortive sneezing. Itching and tickling in the nose. One or other nostril stuffed up. Acute coryza and hayfever worse from the odour of flowers. Often associated with hay asthma. Sore throat on the left side relieved by warm drinks.

CROUP

Aconite (see page 75, and below)
Effects of fright or exposure to dry cold. The first stages of croup or fever, restless, fear, thirst, worse in the evening, lying on the left side, in a warm room, better from uncovering.

Hepar Sulphuris
Starts with a cold, blocked nose, thin irritating discharge – yellow-green. Sensitive to draughts, irritable, worse in cold dry weather; cough when any part of the body is exposed. Sharp sticking pains (see 'Sore Throats', page 102). Desires sauces, spicy food.

Spongia
Croupy cough, waking out of sleep with a feeling of suffocation, alarm and anxiety. Cough worse on talking, swallowing or lying with the head low, lying on the right side; better from lying on the left side.

FEVERS, COUGHS AND CHEST INFECTIONS

Aconite
Most useful in the early stages of any fever or chill, particularly if this follows exposure to dry cold air or a frosty day. It is also indicated when a patient has had a bad fright or shock.

The onset of symptoms is sudden and usually accompanied by fear, restlessness and anxiety; a child with a sudden fever, with a very red throat, burning dryness of the mouth and thirst for cold drinks. The symptoms are worse in the evening, in a warm room or lying on the left side, and the patient wants to throw off the bedclothes. The eyes are suffused, the pulse bounding, but the pupils not dilated. The suddenness of onset and fear are the chief characteristics, but it will often abort a cold or sore throat if given early enough.

Antimonium Tartaricum
This is often a remedy for extreme cases of pneumonia, capillary bronchitis or left heart failure. The patient is bluish, pale, cold and sweaty, but dislikes stuffiness or being wrapped up. The tongue is dry and white but without thirst (Pulsatilla, Gelsemium). There is rattling of mucus up and down the bronchial tree, with a feeling of oppression or suffocation – this rattling is a leading indication for the remedy. (See also Ipecacuanha.) He may be stuporous but want to sit up, and there is a lack of reaction.

Belladonna
The features which suggest this remedy are those associated with overdose of atropine, or the typical scarlet fever picture.

There is a high fever often accompanied by delirium, clouded sensorium, bounding pulse, with twitching and jerking, flushed dry face, circumoral pallor, dilated pupils, dry red throat and exudate with raised papillae on the tongue, and sometimes a scarlatiniform rash. In this case the patient is better from warmth and dislikes being uncovered – the opposite of Aconite. There is frequently a throbbing headache, worse from light, jar, being disturbed, and better from pressure, wrapping up the head. Belladonna may also be indicated for a headache of this type without a fever.

The patient may be in the early stages of tonsillitis or otitis media (the drum may in fact be red), or the start of an infectious fever. If the symptoms are as described, this remedy will often stop the condition developing.

Local inflammatory states with red, hot, swollen, dry appearance are also helped. More toxic than Aconite.

Bryonia
The characteristics of this remedy are stitching pains worse from any movement, dryness of mucous membranes, and desire for large cold drinks. The aggravation from movement may apply to the pain of a pleurisy or pneumonia, to a headache or to a rheumatic or neuralgic pain. Pain in the chest is better from pressure and from lying on the affected side.

The patient is irritable, dislikes being moved or disturbed – even babies can demonstrate this symptom. The mouth and lips are dry, the tongue white, and thirst is present for large cold drinks. There is often a hard dry cough, which is painful and may cause stitching pain in the chest, or headache. The symptoms and signs are frequently more marked on the right side.

Bryonia is helpful in certain cases of measles where the rash is slow to develop, and after which the patient generally feels better.

Carbo Vegetabilis
Characteristically the remedy for collapse or faint, with cold extremities, sweat and blue appearance, but wanting to be fanned or have the window open to get fresh air.

Also of value in capillary bronchitis, with burning in the chest, chilliness, and sometimes spasmodic cough, which makes the patient red in the face (whooping cough). Dry tongue with yellow coating and a good deal of flatulence.

Causticum
This remedy is frequently indicated in laryngitis and tracheitis, after exposure to cold frosty weather and dry cold wind.

Hoarseness worse in the morning. (Phosphorus is worse in the evening.)

Burning rawness down the trachea, with loss of voice. Inability to raise sputum, which slips back. Cough relieved by sips of cold water. Urine spurts on coughing.

These patients tend to be sallow and sickly-looking, and are often irritable, weepy, despairing and full of fears and apprehension.

Ferrum Phosphoricum
Early stages of inflammatory disease, especially respiratory, with fever, deep substernal soreness and painful laryngo-tracheal cough and epistaxis. There is alternating flush or pallor, for no apparent reason, and often an intolerance of eggs. They are more alert than Belladonna, do not have dilated pupils and have a thready weak pulse. This remedy does not have the restless anxiety of Aconite, the burning of Belladonna or the intense thirst of Phosphorus. It is indicated where the symptoms are more obviously respiratory, rather than for a simple sore throat.

Ipecacuanha
Sudden onset of respiratory infection or asthma, with rattling mucus or wheezing. *Nausea*, usually with a clean tongue, spasmodic cough with vomiting. Epistaxis and bloodstained sputum.

Kali Carbonicum
This remedy is valuable in acute chest infection, or in asthmatic or chronic bronchitis.

The patient is chilly and the pains are stitching, knife-like in character, worse at rest, from cold, pressure or lying on the affected side, and the surface is sensitive to pressure and touch. (Bryonia is better from rest and pressure.)

There is a characteristic 3 a.m. aggravation, the asthmatic patient waking at this hour and leaning forward to obtain relief. The Kali Carb. patient does not like the cold drinks of a Phosphorus patient. There is a lot of flatulence and belching of wind. There is the weakness which is present in all the Kali salts. They are irritable, sensitive, drab, uninteresting people, full of fears of the future, of death and ghosts.

Natrum Sulphuricum

A remedy with aggravation from damp weather or warm, damp atmosphere.

The cough is loose with greenish sputum, soreness and great pain, especially in the left lower chest. There is a 4 a.m. aggravation of symptoms, although morning aggravation with depression and diarrhoea after rising are also present. These patients are depressed and may suffer from headaches, particularly following a head injury.

Phosphorus

This remedy is invaluable in the early stages of pneumonia or bronchitis. The patient is restless, nervous, fearful of the dark or being left alone. He wants company and the reassurance of someone holding his hand. There is tightness of the chest with a hard painful cough, aggravated by cold air or laughing, sputum which is beginning to be bloodstained, and a marked thirst for large cold or iced drinks. Notice here the difference in the mental state of Bryonia and Phosphorus – the one irritable and resenting interference, the other fearful and anxious and wanting company. Although thirsty, the Phosphorus patient is often sick, bringing up the drinks a short time after swallowing them. Again, the right lower lobe is often affected, and the patient cannot lie on the left side.

The physical appearance of the patient may also be a guide in selecting this remedy – either slim with brown eyes and long eyelashes, or else red-haired with freckles.

Pulsatilla

This remedy is most useful in catarrhal conditions, recurring colds, sinusitis and asthma; it is also a good acute remedy in respiratory illness, if the symptoms indicate. There is a characteristic absence of thirst, even when the patient is fevered. (See also Gelsemium, Apis.)

The cough tends to be worse in the evening, dry during the night and loose in the daytime, with yellow nasal catarrh or sputum. The patient dislikes a hot atmosphere and the cough is also worse in a warm room. The eyes may be sticky and sore, sometimes with styes or blepharitis – this is frequently seen in cases of measles, where Pulsatilla is most valuable. It will not necessarily abort the measles, but it will hasten recovery with fewer complications of ear or chest.

These patients are weepy and want attention, although they are often jealous when others in the family receive attention.

Appearance may be helpful here, too – the fair haired, blue eyed, rather shy person.

INFLUENZA

Baptisia

Severe flu and even pneumonia, typhoid states with high fever and rapid progression to a stuporous state. There is a red or dusky complexion and the mouth is often coated and offensive (like Mercurius). Gastric symptoms are common with diarrhoea, vomiting and great prostration. Again there is a sore bruised feeling and the patient may complain of his limbs being 'scattered about'. Intense thirst and profuse sweat may also occur.

Eupatorium Perfoliatum

The chief characteristic in this type of flu is the intense bone pains, as if they were broken. The patient hardly dares to move because of the pain (quite unlike Pyrogen). There is bursting headache worse on movement, soreness of the eyeballs, and shivers and chills in the back. There may be bilious vomiting and usually marked thirst (unlike Gelsemium).

Gelsemium

This is the most frequently used flu remedy, particularly in epidemics occurring in mild damp weather. The onset is slow, with aching in the muscles and stiffness in the cervical region. There is extreme weakness, trembling of the limbs and apathy; benumbed. Shivers and chills run up and down the spine, there is a dull headache in the forehead and occiput, with pain in the eyeballs and even ptosis and double vision. The tongue is dirty, but there is absence of thirst even during fever (Pulsatilla, Apis). The patient feels better in the open air and after urination – he may pass large quantities of pale urine, which relieves the headache. He is apprehensive.

Pyrogen

Flu cases requiring this remedy are characterised by extreme restlessness and violent pulsations. The pulse may be fast with a low fever, or there may be a high temperature with a slow pulse. This dissociation is often an indication for Pyrogen. Extreme chilliness occurs, with chills in the back and limbs. The patient feels bruised and beaten and the bed feels hard, bursting headache, and above all inability to be still with the pains and restless feeling. Pyrogen is also a remedy for septic fevers and certain cases of pneumonia.

Rhus Toxicodendron

Although often thought of for cases of rheumatism, this remedy has a definite place in the treatment of influenza. The aches and pains of Rhus Tox. are characteristically worse when the limbs or body are kept still, and improve on moving them, although after a short time the patient becomes tired and stops. The restlessness then comes on again. There is stiffness on first moving or in the morning.

Damp cold weather aggravates the symptoms. There is fever, thirst, redness of the tip of the tongue and aching in the bones in flu. In the confused toxic state, the patient may fear he is being poisoned.

SORE THROATS

Baryta Carbonica

Sore throat occurring after getting the feet wet, recurring tonsillitis with persistently enlarged glands. There is a raw, scraping or shooting pain, aggravated by empty swallowing. Chilliness with offensive foot sweat, salivation, hoarseness and foul taste. The patient tends to be soft, flabby and pale. There is often mucus in the nose and throat and noises in the ears, worse on chewing and better from lying down.

Belladonna

Sudden onset of sore throat with red, inflamed appearance, strawberry tongue and the accompanying dry flush, circumoral pallor. The pupils are dilated and the fauces are dry with difficulty in swallowing. In children the fever may be accompanied by delirium and hallucinations.

Hepar Sulphuris

These cases have offensive discharge and profuse sweating, night and day. The throat symptoms are characterised by a splinter-like pain, as if a fish bone were sticking in the throat, and sensitivity to touch. This sensitiveness applies to any septic lesion in the Hepar case. He is usually also sensitive mentally – irritable, impetuous, angry, made worse by a word, a touch, a breath of air or pain. There is a general aggravation in dry cold and amelioration in wet weather, and a liking for pickles, vinegar and often fat food.

Lachesis

Sore throat on the left side, or beginning on the left and moving to the right, again extremely sensitive to touch, worse from a hot drink and better from cold. Congested blue appearance of the throat, with dislike of any constriction round the neck. Swallowing liquids or empty swallowing is more difficult than swallowing solids. Marked aggravation after sleep. In fever the patient may be loquacious or drowsy, with suspicion of being poisoned.

Lycopodium
Useful in right-sided sore throats better from warm drinks. The patient is typically anxious with a worried frown.

Mercurius Solubilis
To prescribe this remedy in sore throat, the mouth must be dirty, offensive and moist, the tongue being coated with the imprint of the teeth round the edge. Drenching sweats without relief, worse at night and from the heat of the bed, are characteristic. Creeping chilliness is present and, although salivating, he is still thirsty. Mucopurulent discharge from the nose with rawness of the nostrils.

Phytolacca
The throat here is dry, rough, congested and dark red. On swallowing, the pains shoot upwards to the ears like electric shocks. There may be ulceration of the throat and the pain is aggravated by hot food or drink. There is a general aggravation of all symptoms from cold, damp cold weather and at night. The neck is often stiff and there may be an irresistible inclination to bite the teeth together.

The five following *infectious fevers* may usefully be considered here.

CHICKENPOX
Antimonium Tartaricum
Where spots are slow to come out, and especially if bronchitis is present (see pages 97 and 129).

Rhus Toxicodendron
Vesicular eruptions with marked itching.

MEASLES
Consider **Pulsatilla, Euphrasia, Sulphur**.
Bryonia – if you suspect he is incubating it – is fevered and coughing, but the rash has not yet appeared.
Morbillinum (the nosode) after the acute phase is past.

MUMPS

Mercurius: with salivation, offensive sweat.
Pilocarpine: almost a specific remedy in mumps.
Pulsatilla: with orchitis present.

WHOOPING COUGH

Carbo Vegetabilis
Already mentioned (see page 98).

Drosera
The most commonly indicated remedy, with spasmodic cough and vomiting worse after midnight. Also of value in tuberculous conditions.

Cuprum Metallicum
Where spasms are extreme and may lead to convulsions.

Pertussin (the nosode)
To be used either as a prophylactic for other members of the household, or as a follow-up remedy after the acute phase, where cough persists.

GLANDULAR FEVER

There is no specific homoeopathic remedy for this condition, but patients present with fever, rash, small glands in the neck, and often a very painful throat with inflammation and exudate. Remedies to consider are **Belladonna** in the early stage, and **Mercurius Cyanatus** or **Solubilis** if the mouth is dirty with salivation, bad breath and sweating. **Calc. Phos.** can be helpful to follow, for the glands, and a dose of **Glandular Fever Nosode** 30c will often help the rather slow convalescence. **Ailanthus** and **Carcinosin** are also recommended where recovery is slow.

TEETHING

Chamomilla
This is a remedy no doctor should be without in acute illness, especially in children. The child is irritable, wanting to be carried about, or bounced up and down. Whenever he is put down he starts to roar again. Teething, one cheek bright red. Dry cough in sleep. Burning hot feet. Stools often green and offensive, with colic.

Chapter 13

The Cardiovascular System

Many homoeopathic doctors use some of the conventional cardiac drugs in certain situations, but whenever possible these should always be supplementary to a homoeopathic remedy.

In cardiac failure, drugs such as digoxin or diuretics may be needed. We are all aware now of the need to restrict the dosage of digitalis, especially in the elderly, because of toxic effects, and there are some patients who genuinely cannot tolerate any of the cardiac glycosides. Remedies such as Apis, Crataegus and Convallaria may have sufficient diuretic effect, but may need to be supplemented by frusemide, bendrofluazide or aldactone.

In hypertension, diuretic or beta-blocking drugs may be required if adequate response is not obtained by remedies like Crataegus, or by constitutional prescribing.

In angina and myocardial ischaemia there are a number of effective homoeopathic remedies, although, in an acute infarction, intensive care and resuscitation procedure may be life-saving. Aconite, Carbo Veg. and Arsenicum Album can have dramatic effects in acute situations.

In more chronic states, again, look at the patient as a whole. Take into account his general symptoms, his emotional and mental symptoms as well as his pain, breathlessness or oedema, and try to select a remedy covering as wide a range of symptoms as possible.

TINCTURES

Adonis Vernalis
After rheumatism or influenza with valvular disease. Low vitality, weak heart, slow weak pulse. Cardiac asthma. Irregular heart – a possible substitute for digitalis.

Convallaria Majalis (Lily of the valley)
Dilatation of the ventricles – oedema. Sensation as if heart stops and starts.

Crataegus Oxyacantha (5 drops t.d.s. in water)
For weak or irregular heart. Arteriosclerosis and chronic cardiac states.
Myocarditis, worse in a warm room, better in the fresh air.

Iberis (Tincture of 1x potency)
Palpitation from slightest exertion, laughing or coughing – darting pains
in heart. Worse on lying down, on left side, exertion, warm room.

ANGINA

Cactus
Constriction, squeezing of heart. Sensation that an iron band prevents the
heart moving. Violent irregular beats, worse lying, especially on left side.
Hot, sweaty. Fear and distress worse at 11 a.m. or 11 p.m.

Kalmia
Violent palpitations with faint feelings, or slow feeble pulse.
Wandering rheumatic pains in the heart and left arm.
Heart disease resulting from rheumatic fever, especially where rheumatic
    symptoms are better and heart symptoms are worse (the wrong
    direction for cure).
Symptoms worse if leaning forward.

Lachesis (Surukuku or bushmaster snake)
Useful in angina or cardiac failure if symptoms match.
The main characteristics of this remedy are blueness of appearance or
    local lesions, aggravation of symptoms after sleep, tendency to left-
    sided symptoms, aggravation from heat, and palpitation and symptoms
    of choking, out of proportion to the local signs.
Choking feeling is aggravated by touch, hot drinks, empty swallowing.
These patients are often loquacious, jealous and suspicious.

Latrodectus Mactans
Violent precordial pains extending to the left arm and fingers, with
    numbness – radiating to the abdomen. *Cramping* in quality.
Quick, thready pulse.
Anxiety, cold sweat, gasping respiration.
May yell with pain.

Lilium Tigrinum
Dull gripping pain in chest and right arm, worse from consolation,
    warmth, lying down and pressure. As if heart was grasped violently and

then slowly released – wakes her.

Violent palpitation.

Weepy, *hurried*, bearing down like Sepia.

Lycopus (In potency or tincture)

Paroxysmal tachycardia. *Protruding* eyes, *goitre*. Tumultuous sensation in
cardiac region.

Pale, restless. Throbbing worse lying on the *right* side.

Naja (Cobra)

Tremblings worse from sleep, tight things (Lachesis).

Choking, grasping sensation of the throat – irritating dry cough.

Oedema, but *not* haemorrhage or purpura. Surging of blood upwards.

Nerve lesions, even bulbar palsy – paralysis of speech, swallowing with
marked salivation.

Broods over imaginary problems, suicidal depression, dreads to be left
alone.

Pain in the left temple and left orbital region extending to the occiput, with
nausea and vomiting.

Violence of heart beat – audible; valvular lesions, cannot lie on the left
side. Weight on the heart. Stitching pain with *numbness* of the left arm
and hand.

Angina extending to the nape of the neck and left arm, with anxiety and
fear.

Cold body but head hot; worse in warm room; slow, weak, irregular pulse.

Endocarditis and myocarditis. Dull aching pain in back in cardiac cases.

Also hay fever, raw larynx and trachea and even asthma, especially
cardiac.

Oxalic Acid

Severe pain, sharp, lancinating, extending through to the back on the left
side. Worse on movement.

Mottled appearance. Dyspnoea – sharp pain on breathing.

Spigelia

Violent beating of the heart – so that he can hear the pulsation, see the
beats.

Palpitation, worse on sitting down and leaning forwards.

Must lie on the right side with head very high.

Stitching pains, worse from motion. Pericarditis.

Left orbital stabbing pain.

Spongia

Oppression with cardiac pain worse if lying with head *low*.

Constriction, palpitation – sudden waking with suffocation, alarm and anxiety – sweaty. Sensation as if heart is swelling and would burst.

Barking cough.

HEART FAILURE

Ammonium Carbonicum

Pale, worse in cold wet weather, better in dry weather.

Want of energy, power, strength and tone.

Played out – mind and body (after serious illness or flu).

Uneasiness, anxiety, weakness.

Often women; nervous, venous and lymphatic constitution, fat, flabby.

Oppressive fullness in forehead, worse from cold. Nosebleeds on waking in morning.

Coryza with obstructed airways, worse at night.

Emphysema and bronchitis – mucus and rattling like Antimonium Tart.

Asthma worse in a *warm* room, 3 a.m.

Heart dilated – breathless and palpitation on exertion, worse in a hot room.

Faintness with hysteria (nasal effect of ammonia).

Also audible pulsation with great prostration.

Stomach fullness, worse while or after eating.

Acrid fluids – nose, saliva, stool, leucorrhoea.

Antimonium Tartaricum

This remedy, mentioned under respiratory remedies, is the one to think of in acute left heart failure. Accumulation of mucus in the bronchial passages, with rattling respiration and inability to expectorate. Worse from heat.

Patient is pale, or cyanosed, cold, drowsy, and has intense nausea with prostration.

Apis (Obtained from the whole bee)

Of value in oedema and heart failure.

Affects skin, mucous membranes, but also meninges, pericardium. Swelling, stinging, burning, redness, oedema, urticaria. Worse from *heat*, after sleep. Better from cold air, cold applications.

Sudden onset. Puffy eyelids.

Thirstless, even in oedema or fever.

Throat oedematous, worse from heat – may be painless or stinging, burning.

Mind. Sad, tearful, depressed, constant weeping, no sleep from worrying. Irritable, suspicious and jealous. Joyless, indifference.

Fear of death. Restless and anxious.

Arnica

Although thought of as an injury remedy, it has a much wider action. Used for the effects of 'injury' after myocardial infarction or cerebrovascular accident.

The patient and his heart are weak and tired.

Aching as if bruised – bed feels too hard.

May say he is fine when in fact he is seriously ill.

Arsenicum Album

For acute cardiac situations with symptoms occurring at midnight or 1 a.m. Sensation of weight, pressure or constriction of the chest.

Anxious, fearful, restless, prostration, with burning pains, thirst for warm drinks, vomiting and diarrhoea.

Very chilly, but wants head cool.

Carbo Vegetabilis

The homoeopathic 'corpse reviver' – a remedy widely used in situations of collapse, faint vasovagal attacks, coronary attacks, cardiac failure.

The patient is collapsed, cold, sweaty and pale, with thin, thready pulse, but gasping and wanting the window opened.

Nose and lower legs particularly cold.

Sluggishness, distended veins with burning sensations, although cold.

Distension and flatulence.

Kali Carbonicum

Has the weakness associated with all potassium salts.

The heart is weak with irregular, intermittent pulse. Always chilly.

Characteristic stitching pains, especially in the chest in heart or lung affections.

Shortness of breath, must sit up, worse at 3 a.m.

Puffiness of the upper eyelids.

Irritable, very sensitive to noise, and full of fears.

Laurocerasus (Distillation of common laurel leaves)

Contains hydrocyanic acid.

Coldness – want of heat, want of reaction, *not* helped by warmth.

Feeble circulation and weak heart, which may be slow or irregular.

Cyanosis of the newborn and in cardiac cases. Cold, clammy feet and legs.

In *warm* room patient breaks out in cold sweat and *feels nauseated*.

Prolonged fainting. Spells of profound sleep.

Gasping for breath. Any effort aggravates the chest pain. Cheyne-Stokes dyspnoea.

Twitching of face or limbs.

Suffocating feeling – *better* from lying down (Psorinum).

Vertigo – must lie down.

Aching pains in frontal bone (as if brain fell forward).

Dryness of tongue.

Drinks roll audibly down to intestines. Pains in lower abdomen, with loose green stools.

Irritating cough of heart cases worse on lying, but constriction of larynx is better from lying.

Paralysis of bladder with either retention or feeble stream and dribbling.

Chapter 14

The Gastrointestinal Tract

In approaching the treatment of this group of diseases, the physician must use his clinical acumen, accurate history-taking and, if indicated, investigations such as barium meal or enema, sigmoidoscopy and endoscopy, to try to establish a diagnosis. Although this may not alter his therapeutic approach in dyspepsia, peptic ulcer, colitis or diverticular disease, it will help to eliminate the possibility of neoplasm or gross ulceration where surgery may be required.

If a patient presents with a perforation, severe haemorrhage, obstruction or acute appendicitis, a surgical opinion should always be sought. Prescribing of homoeopathic injury remedies before and after operation can greatly ease the patient's discomfort and speed recovery, e.g. Arnica, Staphysagria, Carbo Veg. and Calendula.

Diet plays an important role in gastric and bowel disorders, and the use of bran and high roughage diets is of value in diverticular disease and certain kinds of colitis. A gluten-free diet in coeliac disease, or avoidance of certain sugars where there is intolerance, is essential, but remedies will often enable patients to absorb or utilise foods more efficiently.

Treatment of peptic ulcer still presents great problems, although drugs like cimetidine, ranitidine and the liquorice preparations have improved healing. Relapses still occur on discontinuing treatment, and a homoeopathic remedy, by improving the patient's health as a whole, is more likely to effect a cure. Some patients may require surgery.

In gallbladder disease, inflammation responds well to our remedies, but if stones are present with recurring acute attacks of pain and sickness, operation may be needed. Many patients who are a poor operative risk or elderly may live quite comfortably with their stones under homoeopathic care.

In acute situations, parenteral fluids, blood or intravenous feeding should be given on the usual medical indications.

Early diagnosis of neoplasm with surgical removal still offers the best hope of cure, but homoeopathy can greatly improve the patient's health and often keep him comfortable with a minimum of sedation, even in advanced disease.

This section includes remedies that are often of value in dyspepsia, peptic ulcer, colitis, diverticulitis, diarrhoea, piles and constipation.

While these remedies have local symptoms related to stomach and bowel, try to look at the patient as a whole in his general and mental symptoms. This may help you to select the correct remedy.

Tyler's *Pointers to the Common Remedies, Number 2* is a valuable reference book for these conditions. Symptoms related to stomach and bowel will also be found in the pictures of remedies in Section III.

STOMACH REMEDIES

Anacardium Orientale (Juice of the marking nut)
This remedy is often of value in gastric complaints where the pain occurs when the stomach is empty. There is relief from eating for two or three hours, and then pain recurs. (In Nux Vomica the discomfort is worse while digestion is occurring for several hours after eating.)

There is a sensation of a *plug* in the anus, with urge to stool but not sufficient power to carry it out.

Sensation of a hoop or *band* round the affected part.

The other main sphere of action of this remedy is the *mental* one.

Impaired memory; sensation as if he is double – one part seeking to do good and the other evil. A lowering of moral control with irresistible desire to curse, swear or do violence to loved ones; feelings of unreality (Medorrhinum), marked irritability, irresolution or indecision. Full of fears that he is pursued, that something will happen.

Like Rhus Tox. in skin eruptions – itching, vesicular eruptions.

Arsenicum Album
This is a frequently used remedy in acute gastroenteritis with both vomiting and diarrhoea. There is dryness of the tongue with thirst for small drinks, preferably warm. The stools are offensive, frequent, watery, *excoriating* and *burning*, and better from heat. There is prostration after stool, and profuse sweat.

The gastric upset usually follows a chill, cold drinks, fruit, spoiled food, teething or food poisoning. The Arsenicum mental symptoms must be present – prostration, fear and restlessness. This remedy will also work best in an Arsenicum type – extremely tidy, anxious, restless people.

Argentum Nitricum

Overworked, overtired persons with headache, mental exhaustion, marked anticipatory upset leading to diarrhoea, and a constant hurried feeling.

Flatulent dyspepsia and gastric ulcer with considerable wind and distension. Stools are greenish, like chopped spinach.

Dislike of hot atmosphere, stuffy places, crowds and high places.

Pains in abdomen immediately after eating, relieved by vomiting. During the acute phase there is a desire for cold or iced food and drink. Strong liking for sweet food, especially sugar and also salt or strong-tasting foods, but sweet may upset.

The tongue is smooth and red during chronic diarrhoea, but often pale, flabby and dry with gastric upsets.

Carbo Vegetabilis

This is one of the great flatulent remedies (see also China, Lycopodium, Argentum Nit.). The patient feels blown up and distended and is relieved by eructation or passage of flatus. Again, rich food or cold drinks on a hot day upset.

The patient is usually icy cold, sweaty, with coldness of the extremities and nose. He may be faint and looks pale or blue in colour.

There are small, watery, excoriating stools with burning in the rectum and odourless flatus.

Chelidonium

Remedy for gallbladder and liver complaints, jaundice. Fixed pain, dull or sharp under the lower inner angle of the right scapula – in hepatitis, cholecystitis or pneumonia. Bitter taste. Tongue thickly coated, yellow, with imprints of teeth. Pains in right hypochondrium. Pale stools. Desire for hot drink or warm food.

Bilious vomiting with headache aggravated by heat, warm room or warm applications.

Graphites

This remedy is particularly applicable in persons who are pale, overweight, despondent and lacking in energy. They are hesitant and find decisions difficult to make. Unusual stress upsets them.

Chilly patients, but with dislike of stuffy atmospheres. The stomach symptoms are heartburn, eructation, sick feelings, griping pains with faintness and sometimes vomiting of blood. The pains occur about two hours after meals and are relieved by eating, by warm drinks, by milk and by lying down. There is a dislike of sweet foods. Constipation without any urge and then large pale stool with mucus and colic.

Graphites cases very often have a skin lesion or a history of past skin eruptions, or fissure and piles.

Lycopodium

This remedy is useful in dyspepsia and peptic ulcer. There is much heartburn with eructations and pain in the right hypochondrium (duodenal or gallbladder conditions especially). The symptoms tend to be worse in the late afternoon, 4–8 p.m., and distension of the abdomen is a predominant symptom, with desire to loosen the clothes. Patients may feel hungry but are easily filled up after a small quantity of food. There is often considerable wind in the bowel with flatus, and constipation of a spasmodic kind with pain.

There is a strong liking for sweet food and hot drinks, but the headache or skin lesions in these cases are usually better from cold and worse from heat.

This is often the remedy for the intellectual type of patient with a tendency to worry over little things, to lack confidence, although in fact they are perfectly capable when the time comes. There is fear of the dark, of crowds, and of being completely alone, although they like to be on their own, provided there is someone in the next room. Symptoms and signs are very often right-sided in Lycopodium cases.

Natrum Carbonicum

These patients often resemble a Sepia case – pale, sallow, thin, stooped and timid. There is inability to concentrate, depression and dislike of mental effort, and lack of interest in the family. Symptoms often occur as a result of overwork. They are sensitive to noise, light and tastes, although the sense of smell is poor, due possibly to catarrh which is frequent and yellow in colour. Chilly, but worse in extreme heat, exposure to hot sun or electric thunderstorms.

There is a marked intolerance of milk and aggravation from starchy foods, vegetable and fat, causing flatulence and dyspepsia with acid mouthfuls. They like sweet foods and are often greedy and constantly nibbling. Eating helps for a short time – hunger at 5 a.m. or 11 p.m.

Constipation present or greyish diarrhoea when gastric upset: jaundice.

Herpes of the lips and hair margin, and dry skin with cracks at the finger tips.

Nux Vomica

This is one of the most frequently used remedies for gastric upset, particularly when it follows indiscretion of eating or drinking, or the effects of stress or overwork. The patient wakes up with a headache and a bad taste in the morning.

There is much retching with peristaltic movements and distension, usually two to three hours after food – vomiting tends to relieve the symptoms.

Desire for rich and tasty foods, pickles etc., which upset as the patient is usually 'livery'. There may be flushing or fainting while eating.

Constipation is common with incomplete motions and much straining. It is also useful in colicky diarrhoea, with hard lumps with watery motions and mucus such as is found in colitis.

The general and mental symptoms are a useful guide to Nux Vomica. Chilliness, with aggravation from draughts, but a dislike of hot stuffy atmosphere. Sensitivity to smells, noise and pain, and above all irritability and fastidiousness (one of the extremely tidy remedies, like Arsenicum Album).

Phosphorus

This remedy is useful in vomiting, and in haematemesis where there is marked thirst for cold or iced drinks. These are gulped down, and after a short time vomited up again. Burning in stomach, weak empty sensation in the abdomen. Pains better for cold food, ice cream.

Diarrhoea – profuse stool, blood in stools, sphincter relaxed with involuntary stool.

The Phosphorus patient is tall, thin, artistic, with fine dark hair (sometimes red hair), sensitive and full of fears. She prefers cold iced drinks for burning in the stomach. (Arsenicum Alb. prefers small warm drinks.)

Pulsatilla

The Pulsatilla patient is usually gentle, mild and yielding, with tendency to weep and need for affection, although they can be very jealous. They are often plump and fair-haired. Changeableness is a marked symptom. The gastric symptoms are as follows:

Dryness of the mouth with absence of thirst and persistent taste of food, hours after eating. Pains, sickness and diarrhoea occur from taking very cold or iced food or fruit, especially when overheated, but the heartburn and rawness are aggravated by warm food. These patients often like rich food, pastries and sweet things, but they are upset by them. There is a livery tendency – Pulsatilla is valuable in the cyclical vomiting or acidosis of children that is usually aggravated by cream, chocolate or rich food.

The stools are variable, constantly changing. There may either be burning diarrhoea with mucus, worse at night, or else constipation with ineffectual urging, as in Nux Vomica.

There is a general aggravation from hot atmosphere.

BOWEL REMEDIES

Aloes

Like Sulphur, worse from heat, venous congestion.
Large piles, blue, painful, better from cold applications.
Rumbling in abdomen, colic and urge to stool.
Distension, fullness, liver congestion. Eating causes stool.
Yellowish, thin burning stools, with mucus, driving him out of bed. Lack of control.
Headaches worse from heat.

Chamomilla

This is the remedy most commonly associated with teething in children, with irritability and desire to be carried about. It is also useful in diarrhoea with teething. One cheek flushed. Thirst with a coated tongue. Sour vomiting and hot sweat at night. Sensitive to pain.

The stools are green, small, frequent, offensive or like rotten eggs, with mucus. There is redness and puffiness around the anus.

China

This is one of the windy remedies, with distension not relieved by flatulence or passage of flatus. The patient is often pale, cold and weak, but does not want air (opposite of Carbo Veg.). A remedy indicated after loss of fluid (diarrhoea, bleeding, vomiting).

Diarrhoea tends to be worse in the early morning or after midnight, watery, undigested with mucus and flatus. The stool may be either painless or irritating, but not usually burning.

Colic is better from warmth and lying and worse on eating, especially fruit. There is thirst for sour drinks.

Colocynth

Violent griping, twisting *colic* pains in central abdomen; frequent passage of flatus, with relief.

•Stitching pains in the sides. Abdomen greatly distended and painful. The colic makes him double up, and is only relieved by pressing on the abdomen and doubling up. Paroxysms of colic. Frequent urging to stool. Symptoms are often related to previous frustration or anger.

Magnesia Phosphorica

Spasms of *cramp* in the stomach, griping with belching of wind, which does not relieve. (Colocynth is relieved by flatus.)

Flatulent colic, forcing patient to bend double, better from *warmth* and rubbing.

Magnesia Phos. is worse from cold air, cold water, touch, better from heat, warmth, pressure, bending double.

Mercurius Corrosivus

Diarrhoea with slimy, bloody stools, with colic and faintness and marked tenesmus during and after stool, accompanied by creeping chilliness. The other features of Mercurius may be present. Foulness and offensiveness, sweating, thirst and aggravation at night and from the heat of the bed.

Nux Vomica (See 'Stomach', page 115)

Phosphoric Acid

This is a good remedy for summer diarrhoea, again from overeating, fruit or spoiled food.

The patient is pale, easily exhausted and does not want to talk. Marked apathy and indifference. There is thirst and a desire for sour things, and polyuria.

The stools are watery, *painless*, odourless and profuse, sometimes green and accompanied by flatus. There may be rectal prolapse (note the difference from Arsenicum Album). Debilitating and exhausting.

Podophyllum

This is often the diarrhoea of hot weather. The patient appears ill, pale and collapsed and dark under the eyes. There is cold or hot sweat, a coated tongue and bilious vomiting. Cramps occur in the lower limbs and the colic is better from heat and pressure, and worse lying on the back.

The stools are offensive, painless with flatus and spluttering, and may be yellow in colour. Diarrhoea tends to be worse at night or 3–5 a.m., and after food. Prolapse or piles may be present.

Psorinum

Dirty-looking, rough-skinned, offensive-smelling patient, sweating profusely at night.

Sleepless and hungry during the *night*. Lies on the back with arms abducted.

Sensitive to cold air.

Stools are liquid, very dark, horribly *offensive*, with a penetrating odour of rotten eggs. Sudden and frequent evacuations, but no marked pain.

Veratrum Album

Pale, sunken face.

Excessive coldness, cold sweat of the forehead, icy sensation on the vertex.

Extreme thirst for cold or iced drinks.

Copious vomiting and purging with sweat and collapse, and intense nausea.

Paralytic weakness and loss of power.

Violence of reactions to pain, and mania.

Diarrhoea is profuse with perspiration and icy coldness.

CONSTIPATION

Alumina

Inactivity of rectum and bladder. No real desire for stool although bowel loaded, but great straining to pass any motion. Rectum seems paralysed – no strength to expel the stool. Stools hard, knotty with mucus, or soft clay-like and sticky.

Dryness is also a feature of the remedy.

Desire for indigestible things.

This condition may be relieved in some sensitive patients by avoiding aluminium cooking utensils and foil.

Bryonia

Chronic constipation with *no desire*, and accompanied by headache.

Stools dry and hard – much straining to pass.

The characteristics of Bryonia are the aggravation from movement in headache, chest pain, vertigo, cough, abdominal or back pain, thirst and dryness. Irritable on being disturbed.

Calcarea Carbonica

Constipation with no urge. Feels better when constipated, worse if given laxatives.

Stools often light coloured or white.

Sour eructations and vomit.

In a typical pale, flabby, sweaty, cold person.

Nux Vomica

Urging to stool but nothing comes, or else only a small stool with feeling of not being empty.

May have sticking pains in rectum, with piles.

Bright blood with feelings of constriction.

Indigestion and spasmodic colic. Desire for rich and tasty foods, which upset.

Chilly, irritable, fussy, driving personality.

Opium

Almost unconquerable chronic constipation; from inaction or paresis. Obstruction of bowel from faeces. Stool hard, round balls. Faeces protrude and recede. Lack of peristalsis. Extreme drowsiness and even coma. Following cerebrovascular accident. Of value in elderly patients with inability to pass stools – give in 6c potency twice daily for a week or two.

Silica

Hard lumps, much straining and urging. Stool partly protrudes and slips back – inability to expel. Abdominal walls sore with straining. These patients are chilly, with sweaty hands and feet, thin, timid and lacking in confidence.

PILES

Aesculus

This has a feeling of small sticks in the rectum, with dry, hard stools, and pains in the sacral region.

Aloes

See page 116.

Collinsonia
Where there is much bleeding, and obstinate constipation. Congestion in pelvic organs and rectum. Feeling of sharp sticks in rectum.

Muriatic Acid
For sensitive piles better from warmth, with poor muscle control of anus, prolapse and great weakness.

Nitric Acid
More indicated in fissure with knife-like pain shooting up the rectum and remaining long after stool.

Nux Vomica
A common pile remedy with much tenesmus, and following indiscretions of eating. Very irritable (see page 115).

Paeonia
Where the piles are congested and acutely painful.

Sulphur
Frequently indicated with repeated piles, local congestion and other Sulphur indications.

Chapter 15

The Genito-urinary Tract

There are a number of useful homoeopathic remedies for cystitis, retention, incontinence, renal calculi and leucorrhoea. It is important in cystitis or pyelitis to culture the urine. If your remedy does not clear up the infection quickly, especially in younger patients, further investigation or an antibiotic may be required to avoid chronic renal damage. If haematuria is present, pyelography or cystoscopy should be considered to exclude a neoplasm. Stones may require surgical removal, although smaller ones will sometimes pass with the help of a homoeopathic remedy. In elderly men, remedies may help benign prostate enlargement for many years, without operation, but careful clinical examination and investigation is essential to exclude malignancy.

The remedies described here have useful bladder symptoms. Always remember the more general, constitutional symptoms too, as these may help in selecting the correct remedy.

URINARY REMEDIES

Berberis

A great remedy in renal or gallbladder colic – may help the patient to pass a small renal calculus.

Soreness in renal area worse from pressure, jar of walking or in a car, but restless, because the pains are stitching and *radiate* across the back or down the ureter.

Urging and burning in bladder and urethra.

Of value in pale, gouty or rheumatic patients. Pains move about, stitching and stabbing – in joints, in neck, in back, worse on stooping.

Restlessness. Pains and coldness in head. Characteristically radiating pains from one point.

Cantharis

Violent burning, cutting pains in bladder and urethra which get steadily worse. The patient wants something done quickly, may scream, become irritable and even insolent, and delirious in fever. These symptoms are worse in the afternoon, and the pains occur before, during and after micturition. They are accompanied by tenesmus, and only a few drops of urine pass.

Restless and very thirsty; disgust for food.

Also of value in bowel inflammation with blood and mucus, burning and distension and tenesmus (like Mercurius Cor.).

A remedy for erysipelas – red, burning and blistering. Also given by mouth following burns and scalds, with intense pain and blisters. (Urtica lotion locally.)

Causticum

A most valuable cystitis remedy, with acute sensitivity to cold. Great urgency with inability to pass urine, then later, while sitting, involuntary urination without warning. Shooting pains in the rectum when the patient cannot pass urine.

Incontinence on coughing or exertion.

Retention of urine after operations, especially gynaecological – this remedy will often save unnecessary catheterisation.

Aggravation in cold dry winds and frost, causing paralysis, especially of face, raw cough and loss of voice, and rheumatic pains.

Melancholy, anxious, irritable, full of forebodings.

Clematis

Burning sensation at the beginning of urination – this sensation continues in the urethra for a long time after passing urine. Feels as if urethra will close up – a feeling of constriction, and the flow is very slow.

The bladder is seldom quite empty.

Small itchy crusts on the scalp, pustular rash round the loins.

Toothache, unbearable at night – want to draw in cold air or drink cold water.

Dread of being alone and yet dislikes company. Apprehension, weeping and homesick. Irritable and angry.

Sabal Serrulata

Mainly a remedy of value in prostatic enlargement – can be given in 6x potency twice daily over long periods, sometimes enabling older men to do without operation.

These patients also get confused, depressed and irritable, want to be left to die, and get angry at sympathy.

Fear of going to sleep, because of unknown danger.

Bladder feels full – scalding urine and feeling of blockage in the meatus.
Feeling as if testicles are tightly drawn up. Also pains in the head, aching
in temples, especially right, with vertigo. Pains at root of nose extending
up into head, or at base of skull extending down to cervical region.

Sarsaparilla

Pains at the *end* of micturition – urgency, but little passes. Urine flows
more easily on standing than sitting. White, turbid appearance of urine,
with mucus.

Passes gravel or stones.

Also weakness, sluggishness, failure to heal.

Applications of heat improve, but internal heat aggravates (e.g. hot food).

Like Secale, but Secale is better from local cold and uncovering.

Symptoms generally worse from walking, motion, going up and down
stairs.

Terebinth

Burnings.

Drowsiness, even when having pain.

Smooth, red, glazed tongue.

Tinkling sensation in the ears – own voice sounds unnatural and direction
of sounds is disturbed.

Violent burning and cutting pains in the bladder, with smoky, bloody
urine.

Similar pains in abdomen extending from left to right with distension.

Pains in kidneys worse from sitting, better from moving about.

Haemorrhages – ecchymoses, stomach and bowel, kidney and bladder.

GYNAECOLOGICAL REMEDIES

The symptom of leucorrhoea appears in many remedy pictures. The
correct remedy must cover not only the modalities of the discharge, but
also some of the patient's general symptoms.

Hydrastis

This remedy is best known for its catarrhal symptoms, involving
respiratory, gastrointestinal, urinary and genital systems.

The discharges are characteristically *ropy* and viscid.

Leucorrhoea is thick, yellow, and viscid, with soreness, excoriation and
vulva itch.

The other marked symptom of Hydrastis is an empty faint feeling in the stomach with loathing of food, and obstinate constipation with no desire for stool.

Kreosotum

Putrid, excoriating discharges – yellow staining, with violent itching and *burning* pain.

Offensiveness of all discharges.

Also in tooth decay with pain and bad odour.

Bleeding easily from small wounds. Profuse menses with flow heavy on lying down.

Lilium Tigrinum

A hot type of Sepia. Usually fat and fair.

Hot and *hurried*.

Angry and bad-tempered, depressed and silent, and again indifferent to her family. Feels only she can do a particular thing – no one else can.

Exacting – things revolve round her. Fear of going crazy, of what happens after death. Menses irregular, clotting, heavy. Uncontrollable sexual excitement, worse before menses.

Sensation as if the whole of the inside would fall out (like Sepia).

Mercurius Solubilis

Greenish, biting leucorrhoea, with burning and desire to scratch.

Burning and urging to urinate.

Diarrhoea with urging and tenesmus, mucus and blood.

Worse from the *heat* of bed, worse at *night*.

Sweating without relief; dirty moist tongue with thirst and salivation.

Nitric Acid

Itching, burning discharge with splinter-like pains and ulceration.

Offensive, yellowish, bloody.

The severe pains of anal fissure or piles. These patients are *chilly*, depressed, irritable, indifferent, intolerant of sympathy and sensitive to pain, noise, touch or jar.

Profuse sweat of hands and feet.

Desire for *fat* and *salt*.

Warts.

Pulsatilla

One of the polychrest remedies described fully in Section III, although often a female remedy.

Plump, tearful, mild, yielding person who wants sympathy, and yet is jealous and irritable too.

Chilly and yet hates warm stuffy atmosphere. Better in open air, better from slow movement. Changeable. Most discharges in Pulsatilla are bland, although leucorrhoea can be excoriating, thick yellow or green. Menses are often late or absent – may help to start the period in adolescent girls.

Marked sexual excitement in male or female, and yet fear of the opposite sex.

Sepia

This is one of the most commonly used female remedies, with a wide variety of symptoms.

The most characteristic pelvic symptom is the 'bearing down' sensation as if the organs would prolapse – it will help to improve pelvic muscle tone in certain degrees of prolapse, but severe cases will also require operation. Low backache.

Great dryness of vagina and vulva, causing discomfort on walking.

Leucorrhoea gelatinous, yellow or white, burning and excoriating.

A remedy both of heavy irregular menses, or late and absent ones.

Sudden hot flushes with weakness and faint feelings at the menopause.

The classical Sepia person is chilly, sallow, dull, irritable and indifferent to loved ones, but always better from sleep and from exercise, especially dancing, which brings her alive.

DYSMENORRHOEA

Belladonna

Congestion. Pain preceding the flow. Strong sensation of heaviness as if the whole pelvic organs would drop out, but in this remedy this feeling is worse on lying down and better on standing up.

Pains come on suddenly and cease suddenly, worse from jar and touch.

Vagina feels hot and dry, and the pains are cutting.

Menses too early and profuse.

Caulophyllum
Irregular spasmodic pains with bearing down.
Pains extending to groin and thighs.
Normal flow.
Prescribe between periods.
Chilly.
Associated with rheumatic pains in small joints.

Cimicifuga
Spasmodic pain going from side to side of the abdomen and radiating into
the anterior aspect of the thighs.
Pain like labour pains, making the patient double up.
Pain during the period, with scanty flow.
Headache before the period.
Indicated in women with nervous hypersensitivity, depression tendencies.

Magnesia Phosphorica
Severe paroxysmal cramp-like pains which start and end suddenly.
Better from doubling up, warmth and pressure.

Viburnum
Sudden uterine cramps, with pains in the sacral region radiating into the
thighs. Tendency to faint.
Periods delayed, short and light.

MENOPAUSE

In the menopause, with flushings and emotional symptoms, we should
consider remedies like:

Sepia
Lilium Tigrinum
Sulphur
Lachesis, Cenchris and Squid (Dr Blackie)
Natrum Muriaticum
Staphysagria

These are described in more detail in Section III.

Chapter 16

Skin Remedies

The main types of skin disease seen in general practice include the following:

1) Infective: either parasitic – scabies and pediculosis; or septic – boils and abscesses; also shingles.
2) Allergic: in this group we may include familial tendencies manifesting in atopic eczema. Allergy to local irritants, e.g. nickel, detergents, petroleum, washing and bleaching powders; industrial, such as wood shavings, sugar or flour.
3) Dermatitis due to stress.
4) Acne vulgaris and acne rosacea.
5) Psoriasis and other skin eruptions of unknown aetiology.
6) Warts.
7) Other rarer forms of skin disease.

Homoeopathic doctors are frequently faced with many of these conditions, very often after the patient has had various types of local applications, and has ceased to respond or else become allergic to the treatment. Parasitic infections may require local conventional applications.

Occupational hazards, nickel in buckles, clasps and jewellery, and the notorious 'whiter than white' washing powders must be eliminated. Certain foods such as peas, beans, lentils, milk, eggs, wheat flour and shellfish may be causal in eczema. It is often helpful to start a patient on a few days of water only, and then gradually to introduce vegetable and fruit juices, salads, protein and then the possible allergic foods, one at a time. This will provoke an aggravation if the patient is sensitive to particular foods.

There are certain local skin appearances which may guide us to a remedy, but general and mental symptoms are often essential for cure. In the course of this case-taking we may also come upon a psychological reason for the skin lesion. Local signs of value are:

The vesicular eruptions of Rhus Tox.
The cracks and hacks of Petroleum.
The dry cracking with sticky oozing of Graphites.
The redness and intense itch of Sulphur.
The dirty, smelly lesions of Psorinum.

In homoeopathic prescribing, most physicians regard skin diseases as merely external manifestations of a deeper underlying disorder. This applies particularly to eczema, dermatitis and psoriasis. For this reason the homoeopath prefers to treat the patient with an internal remedy, based not only on the skin appearances and local symptoms, but also on the totality of symptoms. Indeed, in many cases a remedy prescribed on the general and mental symptoms may greatly help a skin lesion. It may only be on further careful study of that remedy that skin symptoms are found to be present in the remedy picture.

Local applications of Calendula ointment, simple cream, calamine, zinc and castor oil with a little coal tar may be needed to relieve cracking and itch, but these should be used sparingly. Steroid applications should be avoided whenever possible, as they have a suppressant rather than a curative action. Although valuable in certain acute situations, they cease to be effective after frequent use and may cause side effects locally (and even systemically from absorption).

GENERAL REMEDIES

Alumina
Skin very rough and dry with eruptions which crack, itch, burn and are worse from the warmth of the bed.
There is a general dryness in this remedy, dry mucous membranes, dry cough, dryness in the bowel with constipation.
The patient may look pale, greyish, wrinkled and old.
Chilly, but likes open air. Slowness and paresis.
Slowness of the mind, of comprehension. Despair, feelings of unreality.

Antimonium Crudum
Horny excrescences, callosities, corns, thickened tender soles of the feet.
Nails split. Warts on hands. Redness and inflammation of the eyelids.
Sore corners of mouth. Child cannot bear to be touched – irritable, night terrors.
Greedy, fat people, oversentimental. Nausea and gastric upset from over-indulgence. Tongue milky-white.

Antimonium Tartaricum
One of the best remedies for *pustular* eruptions, impetigo, chickenpox and smallpox.
Pale sickly face with sunken eyes, drowsy, cold sweat.
Intense nausea relieved by vomiting. Thirstless. Coarse, rattling respiration in bronchitis, pneumonia or left heart failure.

Graphites
These patients are often obese, chilly, pale women, with a tendency to be lazy. They may blush easily or have nose bleeding. They are usually sad, despondent and weepy; apprehensive, timid and indecisive – music makes them weep.

Skin symptoms mainly affecting ears, hands and nails, mucous outlets, eyelids, corners of the mouth. Hard, cracked skin or itchy, moist eruptions.
The nails are thick and out of shape.
Cicatrices and scars may be helped by this remedy.
Scaliness and itching of the scalp.
There is crusting, blepharitis and cracks behind the ears. The eruptions ooze a *thick honey-like fluid*. There may be 'cobweb' sensation on the face.
Itchy, moist eruptions on scrotum.

Mezereum
Itching eruptions worse from warmth of fire, at night.
Thick leather-like crust on the scalp, with pus beneath.
The burning and itching of the eruptions is violent – must scratch.
Neuralgic pains also violent, especially in the face and jaw and following herpes zoster.
Twitchings of muscles and eyelids.
Craves fat ham.
Constant desire to eat.
Despondent and hypochondriacal from the pain or eruption.

Petroleum
Patient is hot but skin feels cold in spots.

Skin symptoms are cracked, fissured palms or tips of fingers, with bleeding eruptions and *thin watery oozing*. Groin eruptions, worse in *winter*.
Redness, inflammation of the eyes with cracks on the lids and great itching. Painful and itching chilblains, worse in cold weather.

Vesicles which break and form yellow crusts; itchy, burning vesicles of the genitals. (Rhus Tox.)
Occipital headache, vertigo, nausea worse in a boat or car. (A great seasickness remedy.)
Pains in stomach better from eating.
Diarrhoea preceded by colic – in the daytime.

Psorinum

Sometimes regarded as a chilly Sulphur.
Rough, dry, cracking skin which looks dirty; rawness, itching and bleeding worse from bathing, worse from warmth of bed.
The patient is very *chilly* but the skin wants air.
Offensive discharges and eruptions with watery oozing.
Hair is dry and lustreless.
These patients lack the ability to heal, are cold and yet have night sweats.
They are mentally despairing and hopeless.

Rhus Toxicodendron

Vesicular eruptions, burning, itching, sometimes pustular and like erysipelas.
Inflammation of the eyelids, with swelling and agglutination.
Blistering eruptions may occur on any part of the body, especially the genital area.
A good shingles remedy.
Restlessness – never at ease, must move.
Characteristic rheumatic pains worse from cold and wet, better from movement.

Sulphur

This is one of the commonest and most valuable skin remedies.

The eruptions are characteristically burning and itching, with redness. The body orifices are red – lips, nose, ears, anus, often with excoriating discharge. The eyelids are often red, with blepharitis. Septic lesions and boils are frequent. The skin lesions are aggravated by heat and after washing.

These patients are either lean, lank and philosophical, or stout with high colour, redness of the face and coarse hair. They are usually untidy and dislike washing. However, do not be put off by a tidy Sulphur, where other symptoms fit.

General aggravation from heat and bath, with hot feet.

They usually feel empty mid-morning, and have a liking for sweet and tasty food, particularly fat and butter.

Morning diarrhoea occurs and the patient hates the smell of his stool, although is not fussy in other ways.

ACNE

This condition, predominantly found in adolescents, is sometimes most persistent, embarrassing and disfiguring. Tetracycline is still the mainstay in conventional treatment, and does improve some cases. Homoeopathy can also be of value.

Calcarea Sulphurica

This remedy is often of help given in 6c or 6x tablets twice daily over several weeks, and sometimes combined with a few doses of a high potency remedy suitable to the patient as a whole. The patient is usually cold, irritable and anxious about the future or his health. Headaches and bone pains are better from heat.

Pimples and abscesses, burning and itching.

Offensive discharge from ears. Also useful in ischiorectal abscesses.

Hepar Sulphuris

Much sepsis, inflamed, tender, better from local heat.

Chilly, sensitive to draughts, sour sweats.

Kali Bromatum

The bromine element, as one would expect, makes it useful in acne.

Fat, fair, lethargic, depressed, sleepy. Restless feet. Worry about themselves – not getting on well at school. Sensitive in case they are backward.

Coarse skin. *Severe acne* worse before menses. 2 a.m. itching.

Hot, aggravation heat and summer.

Sulphur, **Silica** and **Natrum Muriaticum** (with its greasy skin and eruption along the hair margin) may all be indicated, depending on the patient's general symptoms.

Any of the well-known polychrest remedies may be required to deal with a skin condition. Always prescribe for the patient as a whole, and not just for the local manifestations of his disease.

BOILS AND ABSCESSES

Belladonna
In the early stage of infection, where the lesion is hot, throbbing and worse from touch, pressure or jarring.

Hepar Sulphuris
Inflamed, very sensitive, septic lesions, better from local heat, worse from pressure. The patient is oversensitive mentally and physically, irritable and even violent. Give the 10M potency every two hours until relief, or for a maximum of six doses.

Silica
A more chronic septic lesion. This remedy helps abscesses to discharge, and promotes suppuration and discharge of splinters and foreign bodies. The patient is chilly and sweaty.

Sulphur
Recurring spots and septic lesions, often associated with skin eruptions, with heat and itching, aggravated by heat, in a hot hungry patient.

Tarentula Cubensis
Carbuncles, large abscesses with several heads, burning and bluish in appearance.

Dosage
All these remedies should be given in 30c or higher potency, and every two to four hours for several doses, depending on severity, for a maximum of six doses.

SHINGLES

Arsenicum Album
Burning eruption, better from local heat.
Chilliness, restlessness, anxiety, midnight aggravation.

Lachesis
Bluish eruption, often left-sided, very sensitive to touch, better from local cold.
Hot patient with palpitations, choking, loquacity.

Mezereum
Already mentioned (see page 129).

Ranunculus Bulbosus
Frequently used in herpes zoster.

Stitching intercostal pains with great sensitivity, in both herpes and rheumatic conditions, pleurodynia aggravated by cold air, touch. Blue or transparent blisters which burn and leak serum, either round the chest wall or in supraorbital region.

Rhus Toxicodendron
Vesicular eruptions, great restlessness, burning, itching, must scratch.

Variolinum (The smallpox nosode)
May be of help in post-herpetic neuralgia.

Chapter 17

Rheumatic and Arthritic Conditions

This group of illnesses accounts for a large amount of disability and loss of working days. It includes a wide variety of ailments, from simple muscular rheumatism to severe arthritis, and covers some neuralgic conditions and diseases like gout, polymyalgia rheumatica, systemic lupus erythematosis, psoriatic arthritis and connective tissue disorders.

It is important if possible to make an accurate diagnosis from the point of view of prognosis, and occasionally to select a steroid for a condition like temporal arteritis, with its risk of blindness. Apart from this, the homoeopath must look again at the patient as a whole, with emphasis on causative factors, onset of illness, and the patient's general make-up and emotional reactions, as well as the modalities of the local pain.

Sometimes the patient is so preoccupied by his pain and disability that it is difficult to see an overall picture. We may have to palliate with more local remedies initially, until a broad, deep-acting remedy can be seen clearly. We cannot expect to reverse conditions with gross pathological change, such as severe rheumatoid arthritis, but we can still sometimes arrest the process and improve mobility and quality of life. Surgery now plays an important part in some of these.

Analgesics and anti-rheumatic drugs may be necessary to alleviate pain, but they have their own problems of allergy and toxicity. The minimum should be used to allow a clear prescribing picture to emerge, so that a more curative remedy may be found.

Modalities
Certain modalities can be quite a help in selecting a remedy.

Worse from warmth: Bryonia, Ledum, Phosphorus, Phytolacca, Pulsatilla, Thuja.
Better in cool: Ledum, Pulsatilla.
Better in warmth: Arsenicum, Causticum, Colchicum, Colocynth, Lycopodium, Mercurius, Nux Vomica, Rhus Tox., Sulphur.

134

Worse in dry cold: Aconite, Bryonia, Causticum, Hepar Sulph., Nux Vomica.

Worse in wet cold: Arnica, Colchicum, Dulcamara, Rhus Tox., Veratrum, Natrum Sulph.

Better from motion: Chamomilla, Dulcamara, Rhododendron, Rhus Tox., Pulsatilla.

This chapter contains some of the commonest rheumatic remedies. There are others, and in many cases a polychrest or constitutional remedy will have a more lasting effect.

Arnica

The great injury remedy – it helps the effects of shock and bruising. If a history of injury precedes the development of rheumatism or arthritis, always start with a dose of Arnica, even though the injury has occurred a long time before.

Great feeling of weariness, weakness and sensation as if bruised. The pains in the joints are sore and there is a great fear of being touched on account of the pain, especially in gout.

The *bed* feels *hard* to lie on.

Restlessness – must keep changing position. The soreness is improved in a new position.

Irritable, forgetful, but with dreams and imaginings of his accident. Sometimes says he *feels well*, although he is in fact very ill.

Bryonia

In contrast to Rhus Tox., Bryonia symptoms are *aggravated by movement*. This applies not only to joints, but also to headache, and pleural and chest pains. If affects muscles, fibrous tissues and synovia of joints with pain, redness, heat and swelling of effusion, all the symptoms being aggravated by any movement, and relieved by *pressure*, and often by cold. In acute rheumatism there is a heavy sour perspiration.

Other features of Bryonia are dryness of mucous membranes, lips, tongue, mouth, with thirst for large quantities at long intervals, aggravation in dry, cold, east winds, and dislike of being disturbed; irritable and resentful of interference. Despondency and despair of recovery are often present.

Causticum

A remedy of paralysis and contractures. It affects the muscular and fibrous tissues. Indicated in rheumatoid arthritis where there is contracture of tendons, drawing pains, and restlessness at night. Aggravation from *dry* cold, better from warmth, wet.

This relief in wet weather and aggravation in frost is sometimes a leading indication for Causticum.

Stiffness of the neck and Bell's palsy following exposure to cold dry wind or draught.

Weepy, hopeless, despair of recovery, fear of the dark, and that something will happen. Irritable and yet sympathetic to others.

Colchicum Autumnale

This plant flowers in the autumn and also has its characteristic symptoms, diarrhoea and rheumatism, in the autumn. It is known for its use in gout, although it has a wider field of action, and often Ledum is more indicated in gout.

The rheumatic *pains* of Colchicum move from joint to joint, are very sensitive to touch or motion. It affects small joints mainly, and the pain is worse in cold, damp weather, especially in the autumn, and better from heat and wrapping up.

This remedy has certain other symptoms which lead one to think of it. An intense *nausea* at the sight, smell or thought of food, burning and icy coldness in the stomach, and marked tympanitic distension of the abdomen with mucous diarrhoea.

The patients are very chilly and extremely irritable, and oversensitive to external impressions – the pain is unbearable (Chamomilla).

Dulcamara

The characteristic modality of this remedy is aggravation in cold wet weather. Rheumatic pains, catarrh, diarrhoea, urinary troubles and skin lesions – all are worse from cold, wet weather. Pains in the back muscles, above the left hip and in the thighs, better on walking.

Worse in the autumn, rain and cold nights.

The patient with coryza or catarrh wants to be warm, a warm cloth on the face, a warm room.

Diarrhoea with mucus coming on from cold, wet or change to cold weather.

Also warts – large, fleshy.

Ferrum Metallicum

Often indicated in obese, chilly patients who flush easily on excitement. The pains are worse when the limb is at rest and better from *slow* motion (like Pulsatilla), aggravated by rapid motion and better from heat.

The region most affected is the deltoid muscle and the shoulder.

These patients are often anaemic and tired, and have a marked aversion to eggs, with a tendency to vomit at night.

Guaiacum

Chronic rheumatic conditions and gout, with weakness, emaciation and exhaustion, sometimes associated with putrid expectoration found in bronchiectasis or tuberculosis.

Stitching, burning and neuralgic pains worse from *motion* and *heat*.

Pains in the left side of the neck or on one side of the face, in the right shoulder, upper arm and chest muscles. Tearing pains in the right forearm and wrist, the *right thumb* and finger joints, again worse from *heat* and *motion*. Stitching pains around the knees and lower legs with shortening of the hamstrings. Swollen sensation in the limbs, with bone pains.

The patient is thirsty, with aversion to food, hot hands and night sweats.

Kalmia

Affects muscles, tendons, joints and nerves. It is particularly useful where rheumatic complaints are related to previous syphilitic infections, or where cardiac complications have resulted from acute rheumatic fever.

The pains shoot and tear; they change about, wandering down the limbs from shoulder to fingers, or hips to toes, although they tend to go from lower limbs to upper limbs. Motion aggravates the pains, and can also cause vertigo.

Severe bone pains coming on in the night (like Syphilinum).

Neuralgia of the face, or post-herpetic neuralgia, stitching, tearing, cutting and shooting, coming on suddenly and then disappearing equally quickly.

Valvular heart disease of rheumatic origin, with slow pulse, palpitation worse lying on the left side, better lying on the back, when sitting up or bending forward.

Ledum

Chilly person, but pains are characteristically relieved by *cold*.

A remedy for bruising, especially around the eye.

Rheumatic pains tend to begin in the lower limbs and ascend. The right hip and left shoulder are frequently involved. Indicated in pains of the feet and ankles.

Swellings of joints are *pale*.

Gouty states and hard nodosities.

Stiffness of the joints; pain is better from cold and cold applications; worse from warmth of bed at night; worse from motion.

A remedy for puncture wounds. Wounds, abscesses and septic foci are tender but cold and *relieved by cold*, while those of Arsenicum burn and are relieved by heat. Mottled, puffy, bloated face, but cold. (Lachesis hot.)

Phytolacca
Like Mercurius in its throat and mouth symptoms. The rheumatic pains are burning and shooting like electric shocks, worse on motion and during the night, on cold days and in cold damp weather, but worse from the heat of the bed. There is desire to move, but motion aggravates.

Inflammation of fibrous sheaths. Pains particularly in the deltoid attachment and right shoulder joint, with stiffness and aching along the trapezius. Periarticular rheumatism in the temporomandibular joint. Stiff neck with pain on the slightest movement (where Bryonia and Rhus Tox. have failed to help).

A remedy of value in throat infections and in mastitis.

Rhododendron
The rheumatic pains of this remedy are worse in cold, damp weather, windy weather and *thunderstorm*. The patient is generally upset in thundery or stormy weather. Pains are relieved *immediately* on moving, whereas in Rhus Tox. they are first sore and then improved by continued movement. They are better from warmth.

Tearing pains in the neck and back, driving him out of bed.

Pain in the shoulder joint so severe that the arm cannot be moved, relieved by walking about.

Rheumatic headache worse before a storm, better from wrapping up the head.

Neuralgia of the face and teeth.

Also of value in orchitis (Pulsatilla too).

Rhus Toxicodendron
This remedy is one of the most commonly used in rheumatic conditions. It is characterised by aching pains and stiffness in almost any part of the body, in muscle and tendon, but also joints. The pains often come on after over-exertion, and particularly in damp, cold weather.

Pains and stiffness on *first moving* but *relieved by continued movement*, until the patient tires and must rest. They soon begin to ache again, become restless and start to move once more. Pain is better from heat and exercise. Restlessness and aggravated at night.

Ruta

A remedy of injury and sprains – it particularly involves the periosteum and attachments of muscles and tendons, especially at wrists and ankles.

Sciatica worse lying down at night, better in the day.

Sensations of weariness, as from a strain, or a fall or a blow, as if bruised.

Worse from cold and wet, and relieved by motion (like Rhus Tox.)

Its other spheres of action are in the eye, where it helps weak eye muscles or tired eyes, with poor accommodation (not the inflammation of Argentum Nit.), and in the rectum, where it is of value in weakness of muscle and prolapse of the rectum.

Helpful in osteoarthritis which follows an old sprain of the ankle or knee.

Sanguinaria

The rheumatic pains are often in the *right* arm and shoulder, worse at night or turning in bed. Cannot raise the arm. Feeling of lassitude and weakness, not disposed to move or make any mental exertion. Worse in damp weather.

Spigelia

This remedy is especially known for its pains. Hardly a nerve in the body escapes – shooting, burning, tearing, neuralgic pains, particularly in the *eyes, face, neck and shoulders*.

The pains in the eyes are relieved by cold, but all others are better from heat; any movement or jar aggravates.

Mention has already been made of its headaches, shooting over the left eye. Stabbing and neuralgic pains in the eyes, radiating in all directions, with tender eyeballs and disturbances of accommodation.

Stitching pains in the chest from intercostal neuralgia.

In chronic rheumatic diseases such as rheumatoid and osteoarthritis it will often be necessary to seek a broad-acting remedy for the patient as a whole. We must then study remedies like Kali Carb., Pulsatilla, Sulphur, Phosphorus, Natrum Mur., Calcarea Carb., Lycopodium, Sepia, Silica, Thuja and of course the nosodes, particularly Medorrhinum and Tuberculinum.

Chapter 18

Remedies of Depression and Anxiety

In homoeopathy a great many commonly-used remedies have strong mental symptoms. The reader should study these as part of the total remedy picture, as described in Section III and in the larger materia medicas. Also useful is Margaret Tyler's *Pointers to the Common Remedies, Number 6*, in which a large number of remedies are described for use in depression, grief, suicide, insane states, delusions, restlessness, excitement and violence, in loquacity, jealousy and suspicion.

It is important in mentally disturbed patients to elicit physical symptoms, generals, food cravings or aversions, and changes in the mental state from the normal for that patient. (For example, where a normally gentle, affectionate person becomes irritable, violent or suspicious, or an extrovert, friendly person becomes withdrawn, resentful and uncommunicative.) These changes from the normal will often indicate a particular remedy.

In severe psychotic states and schizophrenia it may be wise to seek psychiatric help, or have the patient admitted to a psychiatric unit for their own safety, or that of others.

There are, however, a large number of patients suffering from varying degrees of anxiety and depression who can be helped by homoeopathic remedies, thus reducing or even stopping their conventional tranquillisers and antidepressants, large quantities of which are now prescribed, often with little thought. In taking a patient's history, even for a physical complaint, we often find underlying disturbances of emotion due to past illness, family and social problems, resentments, anger, grief or fright. A quiet, careful history will often allow the doctor to help the patient to a better understanding of his or her symptoms, and advice may be all that is required. However, a homoeopathic remedy covering as much as possible of the symptom picture may make a dramatic improvement in the patient's feeling of well-being and ability to cope.

Polychrest remedies will often work best. We must observe the *indifference*, particularly to loved ones, of Sepia, Phosphorus and

Phosphoric Acid; the marked *irritability* of remedies like Chamomilla and Nux Vomica; the *resentment* so characteristic of Natrum Mur. or Staphysagria; the *lack of confidence* and *anxiety* of Silica or Lycopodium; the *fears* and emotions of Pulsatilla and Phosphorus; the *despair* of Aurum, Psorinum and Natrum Sulph.; and the effects of *fright* of Aconite and Opium; or *grief* of Ignatia and Natrum Mur. Study these broad-acting remedies in Section III and in larger materia medicas to understand the 'essence of feeling' of the remedy in its totality. In post-natal depression, think of Cimicifuga, Natrum Mur., Thuja or Sepia.

DEPRESSION

Aurum Metallicum
Suicidal depression with lack of confidence and irritability and anger from contradiction. Sulky, indisposed to talk, sits apart weeping and meditates on death. Full of self-condemnation but critical of others. Hysteria alternates with the depression, and there is apprehensive fear and terrifying dreams. Discontented with his circumstances and quarrelsome.

Prefers the open air and likes cool applications, but has icy-cold hands and feet.

Calcarea Carbonica
Sometimes considered a slow, sluggish type of patient, but it has all sorts of *fears* in its symptomatology.

Despairs of life, imagines she will die, great uneasiness as if some accident or misfortune will happen.

Dread and anxiety for the future.

Fears of disease or death, that she will lose her reason, that people will observe her confusion, and that they look at her suspiciously.

Easily frightened, especially children, with night terrors and bad dreams.

Sits and fidgets with small things, and broods over things which are unimportant. Obstinate and peevish.

Pale, flabby, sweaty person with cold extremities and sour vomit and stools.

Cimicifuga (Actea Racemosa)
Especially a remedy for women with rheumatic and hysterical symptoms. Depression, anxiety and fear. The fear of death is almost as marked as in Aconite.

Depression is characterised by an awful *gloom*, like a black cloud, and yet mixed with hysterical symptoms and fears of the nature or extent of her illness. *Insomnia* in this type of person. A loquacious, suspicious temperament, will not take medicine in case there is something wrong with it (similar to Lachesis), and like this remedy, valuable in the menopause.

A restless, irritable patient, gloomy but voluble, with flushes frequently colouring a pale face with dark rings under the eyes. Also a remedy with symptoms related to the generative organs, with painful, irregular menstruation, dysmenorrhoea *during* the flow, and left ovarian pain. Mental disturbances in the puerperium, and therefore of value in post-partum depression. (Consider Sepia too, with its loss of interest in loved ones.)

Sensitive; to *cold* and damp, with rheumatic pains, which are better when the mental symptoms are worse.

Headaches especially in the nape of the neck, with pain behind the eyes, relieved by cool open air, and worse from movement.

Drosera

This remedy is predominantly thought of for whooping cough, but it is also a remedy to consider where there is a history of tuberculosis. It has marked mental symptoms in its picture.

Dejected over what others have done to him. Disheartened and concerned about the future. Imagines he has been deceived by spiteful, envious people. Resentful of insults, can become quite enraged over trifles.

Anxiety marked especially in the evening, with desire to end his life by drowning. Dreams of being maltreated. Restless, cannot stick at one thing for any length of time.

Natrum Sulphuricum

A useful remedy where there is a history of head injury, or in patients with asthma or pneumonia, particularly involving the left base of the lung, and occurring in warm wet weather.

Depressed, tearful, with a tendency to weep or feel sad from music (Graphites also). Tired of life but does not really want to end it (whereas Aurum does).

Irritable in the mornings, hates to speak or be spoken to, sensitive to the smallest noise.

4–5 a.m. aggravation.

Phosphoric Acid
The key characteristic of this remedy is its remarkable *indifference* to everything. He does not want anything, does not want to speak, shows no interest in the outside world, cannot collect his thoughts properly. Listless and apathetic.

Ailments from care, grief, chagrin, homesickness or disappointed love, but *without* the sensitivity, hysteria or changes of mood of Ignatia, *without* the intensity and tendency to go to pieces on account of chagrin or resentment seen in Staphysagria. Natrum Mur. is far more intense and passionate, weeps and hates sympathy, whereas Phosphoric Acid has dull apathy in its disappointed love.

Overgrown, overweight children, with growing pains and headaches.

In spite of the prostration running through this remedy there is one contradiction, in that the profuse diarrhoea often seen in Phosphoric Acid does not cause exhaustion, and indeed the patient may feel better after diarrhoea. (Calcarea Carb. is better when constipated.)

Psorinum
This remedy is thought of most often in skin diseases, but it has profound mental symptoms.

A very chilly remedy, with foulness of discharges.

Hopelessness, despair of recovery and fears he will die. Full of fears and forebodings, that he will fail in his business. Dreams of his business.

RESTLESSNESS, VIOLENCE AND DELIRIUM

Arsenicum Album
No group of restless remedies can omit Arsenicum.

Restlessness is a constant symptom, accompanied by *prostration* out of all proportion to the symptoms. *Anxiety* about himself – full of fear, feels it is useless to take medicine as he is sure to die. Extremely fastidious, and sensitive to smells, touch and surroundings.

Together with the chilliness, burnings, and aggravation of symptoms at 1–2 a.m. described elsewhere.

Nash describes Belladonna, Hyoscyamus and Stramonium as remedies particularly indicated in delirium.

Belladonna
This remedy is one of our commonest acute remedies, and has been mentioned in fever, inflammation and headache.

The patient is hot, flushed and dry, with dilated pupils and very dry red throat with constant desire to swallow. *Sudden* onset of symptoms with violence. The child with a high fever has delirium, nightmares, sees animals and ghosts, but the fears and violence are also seen in mentally disturbed patients. There is congestive headache, and the patient is frightened and wants to run away and hide.

Hyoscyamus
Here the patient is pale and weak, often elderly; the low-grade type of delirium predominates with muttering stuporous state, staring at surrounding objects without seeing them, picking at the bedclothes. Now and then violent outbursts occur and the patient becomes restless, getting out of bed and taking off his clothes or talking and singing amorously.

This picture is seen in pneumonia and typhoid states, but also in elderly patients who are confused and in strange surroundings, such as in hospital. They are often very suspicious, imagining that the nurse is trying to poison them, and refusing their medicine. They are also jealous of others (these last two symptoms being seen in Lachesis also). Twitchings of muscles occur all over the body, particularly in the stuporous state.

Stramonium
The wildest and most violent of these three delirious remedies. It resembles Belladonna in the redness of the face and dilated pupils, but above all these patients are *loquacious*. Raving, singing, laughing, swearing or praying. Repeatedly jerking the head up from the pillow, or throwing himself about. Fears being alone and in the dark.

Chapter 19

Remedies in the Elderly

In homoeopathy there are no remedies exclusively for use in the elderly. Any patient may need almost any remedy depending on the total symptom picture, and to some extent the pathology of the condition. Again, polychrest remedies will often be indicated and should always be considered first, but there are some which should be borne in mind for the old and which are easily forgotten.

Potencies can be varied as with other age groups, although it should be remembered that a weak, elderly patient may not have the ability to respond to very high potencies, and may do better on 30c. Some patients with gross pathological change may require 6x or 3x potencies given over quite a long period to alleviate rather than to cure, where this is not possible. However, many old people live an active and alert life to a great age, helped by their homoeopathic remedies. Doctors are now very aware of the care required in giving orthodox drugs to the old, who often react very badly to sedatives, antibiotics, antihypertensives, and certain cardiac remedies, and are better with only small doses, or in many cases no drugs at all. There is no problem such as this with homoeopathic treatment, which is gentle and safe in its action.

A few remedies for the old or those with loss of memory or confusion are considered in this section.

Ambra Grisea
Premature old age. Feeble, trembling, tottering of gait, a dreamy state with forgetfulness. Jumps from one subject to another, asking questions but not waiting for the answer before moving on to another. Alternation of depression with vehemence of temper. Has to make an unusual effort to bring his mind back to concentrate on what he was thinking about. His mind dwells on most disagreeable things and he cannot get rid of them.

Vertigo in old men, so bad that he cannot go out in the street. Symptoms all worse in the mornings. The presence of others aggravates symptoms – this is noticeable in old people who cannot pass a stool in the presence of a nurse or relation, and are often constipated. Also aggravation from conversation, and music seems to be intolerable. Itching in old people.

Anacardium Orientale
This remedy is of value where there is loss of memory, especially in the elderly, but it has a characteristic sensation of dual personality, as if he has two wills in conflict. Everything seems in a dream; has a marked inferiority and worry over his forgetfulness. This applies also to younger patients like students, with fear of failure and anticipation of the ordeal of examinations.

Along with the memory loss there is irritability and desire to curse and swear, sometimes in those with a strict sense of morality or religious faith. This distresses them greatly and causes feelings of guilt. Can be quite malicious. Sensations of a plug in the rectum or ear, or of a band or hoop round a part.

Dyspepsia and pain in the stomach when it is empty, and relieved by eating.

Arnica
This remedy is almost specific for injury or bruising, but it is of value in severe illness or in elderly patients. Old people who get easily tired, or do too much and feel exhausted, will often benefit from a dose of Arnica.

Great weariness and a sensation *as if bruised* is a key indication. This may follow over-exertion or a fall, but also occurs in patients who are in bed a lot or seriously ill, perhaps with cancer. The bed feels hard – he is sore and restless and helped by change of position. (The Arsenicum patient is restless, but anxious and frightened, and not helped by moving; the Rhus Tox. patient must move and is relieved by moving.)

A very *ill* patient may say he *feels well.*

Coldness of the body with hot head.

Irritable, sad, hopeless, indifferent. Does not want to be touched – because of pain; very sensitive even to the approach of a nurse.

Dreadful dreams and imaginings – reliving the events of an accident. Horror of instant death.

Baryta Carbonica
A remedy for slow development in children, but also in degenerative, cardiovascular or cerebral conditions of old age. Enlarged glands and prostatic hypertrophy.

Chilly, pale, withered with weakness.

Premature old age, childish behaviour in the elderly, not clear in his intellect, memory loss, cannot think clearly.

Fear of something going to happen. Hatches up all sorts of complaints and grievances, imaginary worries. Thinking of his troubles makes him worse.

Coarse catarrhal rattling in the chest in old age, particularly in cold, winter weather (Senega, Ammoniacum).

Carbo Vegetabilis

We think of this remedy in faint and collapse, where the patient is cold, pale, sweaty with thready pulse and a desire for air (in heart cases or post-operative collapse). It is also of great value as an old person's remedy, a dose of 30c given at regular intervals, or 6x tablets twice daily.

There is slowness, sluggishness and indifference.

Internal burning sensations but coldness externally, especially feet and legs, hands and nose. Venous sluggishness, blueness, varicose conditions. Much flatulence.

Cocculus

A remedy useful where the patient suffers from the effects of loss of sleep, coupled with anxiety as in nursing a loved one. She is weak, prostrated, cannot sleep or suffers anxious, frightful dreams. There is congestive headache, and vertigo with nausea, with extreme sensitivity to motion. This may occur in Menière's syndrome, cerebral ischaemia or even in travel sickness. There is overwhelming nausea at the thought or smell of food.

Paralytic stiffness of limbs, weakness of the back and legs, of the neck muscles, and numbness of feet and hands. Paralysis of eyelids and throat, and inco-ordination like Gelsemium. Anxious, melancholy, sensitive to insults or disappointment, slow concentration or in answering, cannot find the right word, cannot bear noise or contradiction.

Conium

Progressive weakness of memory, mind becomes tired and he cannot concentrate or stand any mental effort. He is unhappy, indifferent to things, peevish and will sit and mope in a corner. Any kind of excitement brings on physical or mental distress.

Vertigo on turning the head, worse when lying down, worse on moving the eyes and better if the eyes are closed.

Trembling and paralytic symptoms, and a curious symptom where aching in the legs from rheumatism or ulceration is better from allowing the legs to hang down.

Chapter 20

Children's Remedies

While there are certain illnesses more commonly encountered in children in general practice, the basic principles of homoeopathic prescribing remain the same – to find a remedy most suitable to the child as a whole, and having symptoms most similar in its 'drug picture' to those presenting in the patient. In using homoeopathic remedies we can give the same quantity in the same potency at the same intervals, whatever the age, from the newborn to the very elderly, because we are prescribing a stimulus to the patient and not a pharmacological dose. In acute illness, 30c or 10M are most frequently prescribed, and in more chronic conditions, a few doses of 30c will again prove satisfactory.

We believe that a homoeopathic remedy acts in a very small dose because the effect depends on its careful selection for that individual, at that particular time, and because an ill person is sensitive to a small dose which would not affect a healthy person. For that reason, a large quantity of a single potentised remedy, or a mixture of remedies taken at one time, will not normally cause a reaction (whereas repeated doses of a single remedy for some days or weeks may cause the effect of a proving, with aggravation of symptoms). Hence if a child inadvertently finds your medicine case, and swallows the contents of several bottles at once, no untoward effects will result and nothing need be done.

ACUTE CONDITIONS

The commonest ones seen in children are injuries, infectious fevers, and acute respiratory and gastrointestinal complaints. Remedies for these are described in the relevant chapters of this section, the symptom pictures applying equally to adults and children. Here a good knowledge of a few acute remedies like Aconitum, Arnica, Ferrum Phos., Belladonna, Arsenicum Alb., Chamomilla, Pulsatilla, Phosphorus and Sulphur will go a long way to helping most cases. They are safe and rapid in action with no side effects.

CHRONIC CONDITIONS – BORLAND'S FIVE GROUPS

When faced with more chronic problems such as recurrent coughs and colds, allergies, eczema, asthma, bed-wetting, constipation or behaviour problems, try to look for a constitutional prescription for the child rather than his illness.

Dr D. M. Borland was one of the great observers of children, and in his book *Children's Types* he vividly portrays various kinds of children in groups, numbered 1 to 5, giving not only a picture of their symptoms and behaviour, but often comparing one remedy with another. These are by far the best children's studies available in our materia medica, and I make no apology for describing them in an abbreviated form in this chapter. Each of the five groups described contains a set of related remedies. The descriptions of the related remedies follow on naturally one after the other.

Group One is the Calcarea group: Calcarea Carb., Calcarea Phos., Phosphorus, Silica, Lycopodium, Causticum, Tuberculinum.

Group Two is the Baryta Carb. group: Baryta Carb., Borax, Natrum Mur., Sepia, Aurum, Carbo Veg.

Group Three, the Graphites group, contains remedies useful in skin conditions: Graphites, Capsicum, Psorinum, Antimonium Crudum and Petroleum.

Group Four is the Puslatilla group, mostly hot-blooded remedies: Pulsatilla, Suphur, Thuja, Iodine, Fluoric Acid.

Group Five, the Arsenic group, contains nervous and emotional remedies: Arsenicum Alb., Chamomilla, Cina, Magnesia Carb., Ignatia, Zincum.

Calcarea Carbonica (Group 1)

Soft, smooth, smiling baby, with sweaty head. Fat, fair, chilly, lethargic. Lack of energy. Tendency to rickets, big head, slow closure of fontanelles. Although chilly they get hot on the slightest exertion, sweat at night, and may stick their feet out of bed (Pulsatilla, Suphur, Chamomilla). Sluggish mentally and physically, slow at school and at games, weak muscles and ankles. Content to sit and do nothing, clumsy, give up easily, sensitive to criticism or being laughed at.

Scared, especially when unwell or alone, and of going to bed in the dark.

Night terrors and dreams – seeing faces. Aggravation from physical or mental exertion, or rapid motion – car and train sick.

Dislike of too hot food, aversion to meat, craving for eggs, and often for indigestible things – chalk, coal.

Constipation – but tend to be more comfortable this way – laxatives upset them. Stools often pale and diarrhoea if chilled.

Liable to catch colds, tonsils and glands enlarged. In children, this remedy can be given repeatedly, even although the child is improving.

Calcarea Phosphorica (Group 1)

Here the child, while still retaining many of the Calcarea Carb. characteristics, is thinner, with adenoidal tissue and small cervical glands. Brighter at school and definitely growing, often with *pains* in the legs, particularly muscular pains.

Headaches in growing girls, when studying. Dislike of interference. The child is restless, moving about, reluctant to talk, discontented and peevish – always complaining that something is wrong. Indisposition to work, cannot concentrate. Full of vague fears and dreads, especially in the evening. Anxiety causes tummy upsets and diarrhoea – colic in infants after eating – green, slimy hot, watery stools. These children love *tasty* foods, ham rind, kippers. They are upset by ice-cream and cold drinks.

A useful remedy in recurring coughs and colds in growing children.

Phosphorus (Group 1)

Slim, with either reddish hair and freckles, or brown hair and eyes and long eyelashes (like Tuberculinum Bovinum).

Chilly except for head and stomach, which prefer cold.

Sweats, if anxious or on much exertion.

Liable to flush on excitement or with hot food.

Affectionate and likes sympathy and attention, and physical touch, but not so much if very ill – indifference.

If tired or upset can fly into a passion.

Fears – dark, thunder, especially at twilight – sensitive to atmosphere.

Headache better in cold air, prefers to be propped up, and not lying flat.
Hunger before headache.

Desires salty taste, sour, cold – *thirst* for large cold drinks.

Colds start with one blocked nostril, one running – bleeding.

Raw hacking cough worse lying on left side, worse going from hot to cold air, but prefers fresh air, worse on talking.

Right basal lung inflammation.

Silica (Group 1)

Chilly, thin child, with fine hair, light brown. Pale, *sweaty*, especially feet and hands, which are clammy – hands go dead, improved when put in hot water.

Tendency to sepsis, boils, septic cuts or eczema, poor nails.

Lack of strength, easily exhausted by talking and, therefore, dislikes speaking. Shy, lack of confidence, *dread of failure*, over-conscientious, *resentful*, but can be witty and good fun if encouraged.

Likes cold food and drink; milk upsets; hot drink causes sweating.

Headaches: better from heat and warmth, worse from cold, physical or mental exertion.

Lycopodium (Group 1)
Thin child, growing, sallow complexion and thicker skin than Phosphorus.

Chilly, but sensitive to stuffy atmosphere.

Desire for *sweet* foods and *hot* food or drink.

Liable to digestive upsets, good appetite but failure to gain weight. Enlarged abdomen, but not the palpable mesenteric glands of the Calcarea salts.

Headaches from overwork at school, like Calcarea Phos. – a dull ache.

Anxious, *diffident*, lacks assurance, tends to *worry* and become keyed up before events. Liable to bite his nails. Often the worried frown.

Right-sided symptoms.

Aggravation between 4–8 p.m.

Causticum (Group 1)
Sallow appearance, usually thin.

Rheumatic symptoms *better in damp weather*. May get acute muscular rheumatism, particularly from exposure to cold dry wind. Stiffness about the joints and growing pains.

Facial palsy or torticollis developing after exposure to an icy wind.

When overworked or nervously distressed they get chorea symptoms, with jerking persisting during sleep.

Clumsiness and liability to strain muscles (Calcarea – the ankles).

Aversion to sweet foods (opposite of Lycopodium).

Acute thirst after meals, when they have digestive upset.

Sensitive children – to pain and any emotional disturbance – the idea of pain is worse – if they think another child is being hurt, they will cry.

Warts.

Nocturnal enuresis.

Tuberculinum Bovinum (Group 1)
Particularly where there is a family history of tuberculosis. It is usually unwise to give this remedy when the child is actually suffering from tuberculosis in an acute phase.

'Tub.' children are often like the Phosphorus child in appearance, slender, attractive with red lips, brown eyes and dark hair and long beautiful eyelashes. There is often a fine 'down' of hair running down the middle of the back.

A valuable remedy in children with repeated cough, colds or chest infections, usually given as a single dose, between other remedies like Calcarea Phos., Phosphorus or Silica.

Periodicity of symptoms or intermittent fever.
Desire for salt, cold milk. Eats well but remains thin.
Temper tantrums in children. Love of change or travel.

Baryta Carbonica (Group 2)
This is the main remedy to consider in children who are *backward*. They also tend to be small for their age, late in speaking, walking, dentition, gaining weight.

Excessive *shyness*, nervous of strangers, of being left alone, of going out of
   doors and, in a town child, of going into open fields.
Touchy, dislike interference, easily irritated.
Forgetful, never play long with one toy, lack of attention and ability to
   concentrate – this is noticeable in the older child at school.
Any sustained effort exhausts them – they become irritable, and in older
   children this leads to frontal headache.
Chilly and liable to catch colds.
Recurring sore throats and hypertrophied tonsils, enlarged glands.

Also enlarged abdominal glands, poor posture, prominent abdomen. Eating aggravates – touchy, tired and irritable after eating. Constipation.

Crusty skin eruption on the head, crusty eyelids and general upset from washing. (Psorinum has these symptoms and follows well.) The skin eruption may be very irritable, although there is not much to see on the surface.

Borax (Group 2)
Pale, earthy, suffering expression. May be similar in appearance to Baryta Carb. and a bit slow mentally and perhaps undersized, but *frightened*. *Fright* from noise (sudden) – child starts at slightest noise, and from pain. Night terrors, although usually with some cause – child doing too much in the day, or overexcited in the evening – then night terror. Aggravation from *downward motion* – terror. (Lift, or baby being put down.)

Valuable in airsickness (dropping sensation and terror).

Stomatitis – salivation with white spots on the tongue, lips or inside of the cheek.

Herpetic eruptions about the lips, or a generalised herpetic eruption on the body.

Mucous membrane inflammation may cause pain on micturition, without definite infection, and possibly enuresis.

Mentals – inability to learn, from *idleness* – if they would put their hearts into it they could learn. Never settle to anything, even at play they won't stick to anything. Get bored and change from one thing to another.

Much more irritable than Baryta Carb. Irritability ends in passion – kicking and screaming.

Stomach – Acute attacks of diarrhoea and vomiting, particularly colic after fruit.

Borax child gets nausea and sickness from intense concentration; Baryta Carb. gets frontal headache.

Natrum Muriaticum (Group 2)

These children are usually undersized and underweight. They appear shy but really more *resent interference* or being handled, and will burst into tears. They tend to cry more with *rage* than with terror (which the Baryta Carb. child does).

If they are crying, *firmness* helps to settle them, or allowing them just to sit in a corner and watch. Soothing makes them worse. Natrum Mur. children are awkward and knock things over, due to being in a hurry rather than clumsy. They are often slow in learning to speak, and may stammer or have faulty speech due to difficulty in articulation. May be of value in autistic children.

They tend to have thin necks and small, shotty glands at the back of the neck.

Skin eruptions occur at the margin of the hair; there is a greasy appearance of the face, and tendency to acne in teenagers. The tongue has red and white patches which are sensitive, like the mapped tongue in the adult. A tendency to herpes on the lips. The remedy again has pressing frontal headaches over the eyes, especially from study and mental concentration (like Baryta Carb. and Calcarea Phos.).

Chilly children, sensitive to draughts, shivering or sneezing from change of temperature, but also very *sensitive to heat*, stuffiness and exposure to the sun, causing headache.

Salt craving.

Hang-nails, splits at the sides of nails, sensitive and slow to heal.

Sepia (Group 2)

Sallow, greasy skin.

Depressed, moody, sluggish, disinclined to work and even loss of interest in playing. A *negative* attitude to everything. If pushed they will sulk or weep.

Nervous, scared of being alone, of the dark, and yet dislike of being handled (Natrum Mur.). Dislike of going to parties or meeting friends, due to sluggishness, but once they get there they brighten up, and if they *dance* they come alive, and are happy (adults too).

Tendency to nod the head.

Constipation and associated enuresis, usually in the first sleep, before 10 p.m.

Tendency *to faint*, especially in a close atmosphere, standing at school or in church.

Sensitive to *cold* – develops a cold from any change of weather.

Greedy child, upset by milk.

Tendency to sweat; itching of skin without much eruption.

Aurum (Group 2)

Sallow, dispirited, sluggish child – depressed negative attitude.

An undeveloped child – not necessarily small but slow in developing (like Baryta Carb.).

Often boys – undescended testicle.

Lifelessness, miserable and lacking in 'go'; no initiative – everything seems an effort. Backward at school, poor memory, but if contradicted they fly into a rage.

In spite of sluggishness, they are terrified of pain and very sensitive to it. Sensitive to noise, and have acute sense of taste and smell.

Sensitive to disappointment – grieve for days; out of all proportion.

Sobbing in sleep, without waking and without distress the night before.

Catarrh persistent. Infected by hypertrophied tonsils, with offensive secretion in the crypts.

Offensive nasal discharge.

Otitis media with tonsillitis and often purulent, smelly ear discharge.

Carbo Vegetabilis (Group 2)

This remedy picture is not really a type in its own right, but develops as a *result* of a preceding illness, such as measles, bronchitis or pneumonia, influenza or whooping cough.

The child is *sluggish*, dull, lacking in 'go'; easily discouraged, peevish, slow in reacting.

Also sluggish *circulation*. Heavy, sallow complexion with bluish fingers and toes, and coldness of the extremities.

Dull, *occipital headaches*, with inability to work or concentrate. When tired and having headaches he gets violent nightmares, of ghosts, faces.

Although cold and sluggish they are liable to get *hot* and *sweaty* at night, with sour-smelling sweat, generalised, but particularly on the extremities.

Epistaxis.

Digestive upset, with flatulence, constipation and swollen abdomen.

Attacks of diarrhoea, offensive, watery in-between.

Desire for *sweet* things, which upset, and *salt*.

Aversion to *fat* and rich food, which upsets, and *milk*.

Graphites (Group 3)

Fat, heavy pale child with large head and droopy eyelids. Flabby with muscular weakness, easily tired out, sensitive to motion and travel.

Rheumatoid pains affect the neck and lower limbs.

Chilly – like to be covered up but prefer air. Unstable circulation. When excited tend to flush up and even get epistaxis.

Mentally they are timid, miserable and lack assurance; they hesitate in replying and cannot make decisions. Tend to be lazy and averse to work. Although sluggish, lazy and uncertain, they are anxious. Tend to look on the hopeless side, look for trouble, dread new school. Critical. Sensitive to music, which makes them weep.

Skin – most Graphites patients have some skin complaint. Harsh dry skin (unlike the soft sweaty skin of Calcarea). Tendency for fingers to crack and bleed on exposure to cold, or in cold water.

Sticky, yellow oozing discharge. Cracks and discharge behind ears, at corners of mouth and eyes, bends of elbows, groins.

Fissures at anus. Crusts form with gluey discharge underneath.

Chronic otitis with discharge, and the same sticky yellow discharge causing eczema of the external ear.

Nasal discharge and large tonsils.

Blepharitis with sticky eyelids.

Adolescents get acute acne.

Big appetite, upset if empty, better from eating.

Dislike of *sweet* and *fish*.

Attacks of abdominal cramp, relieved by hot milk.

Constipation – feels upset by it, worries over it. Stool may contain stringy mucus.

Sleepy in day – slow to get to sleep.

Capsicum (Cayenne or red pepper) **(Group 3)**
Burnings.
Fat, rather lazy, *obstinate* child with clumsy movements – rarely neat.
    Flabby. Chilly.
Reddish cheeks, or pale and flush up like Graphites.
Sluggish, rather backward with chronic hoarseness and a history of acute
    sore throats – not quinsies, but just acute throats, transitory attacks of
    earache.

Mentals – Forgetful on an errand, partly due to lack of attention. Touchy,
easily offended, easily irritated. Strange dislike of being away from
home – perhaps due to being touchy and lazy and a feeling that they are
not appreciated. They have to make an effort, and can be agreeable when
away – at home they may be unpleasant. Hypersensitive to noise, touch.
Dull, slow at school, poor memory.

Local hyperaemia – in earache the whole ear is bright crimson. In
    rheumatism one joint is affected and has a localised blush over it.
Bright crimson face with enlarged tonsils, *burning heat* in the mouth and
    intense thirst. They want cold drinks during fever, but this makes them
    shiver.
Valuable in *chronic ear discharge* with eczema of the external ear, or
    hyperaesthesia over the mastoid.
Capsicum children often have acute cystitis, *burning*, intense irritable pain
    on urination.

Psorinum (Group 3)
Thin, sickly children, with lack of stamina, easily exhausted by any effort,
physical or mental. Liable to become mentally confused under stress.
Dispirited, hopeless, peevish and irritable.

They look unhealthy, *dirty* and unwashed.
Dry, rough skin, with tendency to smelly sweat.
Skin lesions like Graphites, but with a watery or purulent, offensive
    discharge. *Intense irritation*, worse from *washing*.
Scratches the skin till it bleeds, nearly driven distracted.
Acute blepharitis, purulent nasal discharge, excoriating the lip, and smelly
    otorrhoea.
Abnormal appetite; lack of food causes violent headache.
Useful in hayfever prophylaxis, a single dose in the spring – not in the
    acute phase.

Antimonium Crudum (Group 3)
Overweight, fat, pale children with tendency to redness round the eyes and moist eruption behind the ears.

Mentally these children are a contradiction.
On the one hand irritable, peevish and made worse by soothing (Natrum Mur.). Night terrors.
On the other, impressionable, sensitive, easily upset emotionally, liable to burst into tears from emotional stress, or if their feelings are touched. Under stress they become pale and faint.
Skin eruptions – large, crusty, smelly eruptions – the typical crusty impetigo on the face.
Skin lesions are made much worse by washing (Sulphur, Psorinum), inflamed and painful from radiant heat.
Clumsy, jerky movements.
Warts – numerous, flat, on fingers.
Deformed, thickened nails; also tender thick skin on soles.
Digestive upset from acids, sour fruits or sour drinks.
Tongue soft, flabby and coated *white.*

Petroleum (Group 3)
Again a remedy with skin eruptions, but a thin child with an abnormal appetite, even hungry between meals.
A *seasick* and train-sick remedy, but often with occipital headache accompanying the nausea (which Tabacum does not have).

Irritable, *quarrelsome*, easily offended.
Mentally bright, but lazy, inattentive and forgetful at school.
Sensitive to *noise*, sudden or loud noise – scares them. Nervous of crowds.
Chilly.
Skin eruptions – deep, painful cracks with watery yellow fluid, behind ears, in folds, corners of mouth, anus, groins, axilla.
Sensitive crusts, tendency to bleed.
Itch is most marked in the day (Sulphur at night).
Cracks and *painful bleeding fissures* on fingers.
Liable to *colds*; nose blocked, excoriating discharge, crusts, deafness, otitis with watery discharge, redness and eczema of the ear.
Itchy eyes, blepharitis and lachrymal duct infection.
Bladder irritation, cystitis, raw and smarting; enuresis.
Abdominal colic and diarrhoea on exposure to cold – raw, red anus and perineum.

Pulsatilla (Group 4)

There are two types of Pulsatilla child. One is small, finely built, with fine skin and hair, unstable circulation, liable to flush up from emotion and then go pale; shy, sensitive, affectionate, easy to handle and definitely responsive, bright and lively.

The other, less often remembered, is fatter, with more colour, rather darker hair, more sluggish in reaction, with more tendency to weep, craving for attention, but less responsive. Irritable and slow in the morning.

Sensitive to heat – they flag, lose their energy and sparkle, hang about and get tearful or irritable.

Liable to *digestive upsets* – particularly if *chilled or cold* during a hot spell – they get sick or have diarrhoea, cystitis or earache.

Taking ice-cream in hot weather upsets – rich food upsets, like butter and cream, but they dislike fat.

During fever they get *chilly*, shivery. Often acute colds with coryza, gastric upset, nausea or even vomit. Although chilly their head is better in the open air, worse in a *stuffy room* and there is *bland* nasal discharge.

Conjunctivitis – eyes stream in the open air, sensitive to cold draught; photophobia, itching of eyelids and styes on the lower lid.

Earache – usually from exposure to cold; violent pain spreading over the face, bursting feeling, better from *cold* applications.

Sunset aggravation, nervous with tendency to *nightmares*, fear of the dark and being left alone, yet most lively in the evening and before bed.

Giddiness from looking up at high things.

Sleeps with hands above his head.

Sulphur (Group 4)

There are two types of Sulphur child. The first is of a heavier build, coarse hair, big head, high colour with rough skin and red extremities, hands and feet. Also redness of lips and ears and eyelids, with blepharitis and styes.

The second is thin, with big head and spindly legs, biggish abdomen, paler colour and rough skin, dry with tendency to split or crack. A miserable, seedy child, easily tired, liable to weep; attempts to comfort annoy him. Inability to stand long, irritable if hungry.

Heavier Sulphurs are quarrelsome, impatient, critical, fault-finding and discontented, and lazy, possibly due to tiredness on exertion.

Dislike of interference.

Sluggish, dull and cross, and yet when stimulated they can be *bright* and *interesting*, *friendly* and often clever.

Pleased with their possessions; toys, family, car are all better than others.

Skin irritation – worse in warm and at night. Pleasurable sensation from scratching. Every kind of eruption, intense irritation of all kinds.

Redness of orifices, nose, ears, mouth, urethra, anus.

Heat aggravates but unstable mechanism – waves of heat and chilliness.

Sometimes hot head and cold hands, or hot hands and cold feet – not all Sulphurs have hot feet. Bathing aggravates. They smell – eruptions, discharges, perspiration.

Desire *tasty*, highly seasoned foods, also sweet. Food that is out of the ordinary. Sluggish and sleepy after meals.

Upset by milk, may get diarrhoea. Some children, like adults, like fat.

Usually constipated, with big abdomen.

Terrifying nightmares.

Chronic nasal discharges – offensive, excoriating.

Chronic tonsillitis, infected, hot, offensive breath, masses of glands. Shivering, sweating and thirst in attacks.

Chronic ear discharges, excoriating, pain aggravated by hot applications.

Chest conditions – chilly in a draught, but cannot stand stuffy atmosphere.

Jaundice in children.

Rheumatism, with sweat, heat, red tongue worse from heat, better from movement.

Thuja (Group 4)

The Thuja child tends to be small and finely built, dark or fair. He may be slightly backward, but sometimes the lively, active child gives this impression because he hesitates and finds difficulty in choosing or saying words, and this makes him appear slow.

Disinclined to talk, rather silent. Activity seems to brighten him up, but he becomes dull and heavy if left to sit.

Extremely sensitive, responds to kindness, is easily upset emotionally, conscientious, and in particular *sensitive* to *music* – may even weep from music. Sad and may weep like Pulsatilla. Possibly of value in the autistic child.

Sensitive to the *cold* and damp but better in the open air. Worse in the mornings.

Greasy skin, especially in dark children. Fair children may have down on the back, like Tuberculinum Bovinum.

Sweating on exertion and *sweat* on *being uncovered.*

Neuralgic *headaches* on mental stress, or when overtired or overexcited. These pains may be in localised areas, which are painful and sensitive.

Chronic *catarrh* – thick yellowish-green – crusts in nose, chronic otitis media.

Poor *digestion* – particularly upset by onions, and in older children, by tea.

Gurgling in the abdomen, full boggy caecum with attacks of diarrhoea. Pale, greasy, almost fatty stools with flatus.

Warts – soft, tend to bleed.

Upset from vaccination.

Iodine (Group 4)

Dark-haired, dark-skinned, thin. A bit like the Sulphur child, but without skin problems.

Intense restlessness – fidgeting.

Sensitive to *heat* – room, bath, sun.

Irritability – sudden, impulsive – may strike another, although playing quite happily. Following this they get depressed and silent and lose interest.

Hunger – exhausted if long without a meal, headaches.

Although they eat, they do not gain weight.

Acute nose infection, hot, watery, irritant discharge, sinus pain, sneezing, watering eyes, but nose feels obstructed.

Chronic eustachian catarrh and deafness.

With the cold they get laryngitis, hoarse, painful croup.

Intensely hot dry skin with croup – restless, anxious, like Arsenicum. (But Arsenicum is chilly – Iodine is hot and dry.)

Asthmatic breathing, better in open air.

Diarrhoea attacks – frothy, fatty, whitish stools, perhaps pancreatic in origin.

In children with bright red cheeks you may get acute rheumatism – violent pains better on moving, worse from heat, sharp and stabbing.

Like Bryonia, but it is thirsty, white tongue, more dull and heavy and averse to food. (Iodine – alert, hungry.)

Fluoric Acid (Group 4)
Often fair-haired, thin, fine-boned, a bit like Silica to look at. Sensitive to *heat* – hot room, hot sun, too many clothes. Red sweaty palms, offensive foot sweat but hot and sore. Unhealthy finger nails, brittle, cracked, splintered. Dry and fissured tongue.

Mentals. Yielding disposition, but not very irritable, patient, and enjoyment of life – of the simplest things – cheerful.
   Tired with mental concentration, headaches at school and not very bright at bookwork. *Headaches* also if constipated or having to hold urine for a long time in school. Tendency to make mistakes in writing, to transpose words or letters.

Unreasoning hatred of other child – no cause.
Better from *physical exertion.*
Poor at standing – faint, headachy or tired.
Hunger between meals causes headache; hunger in middle of night. In spite of eating they remain thin, small and fine.
Desire for *highly seasoned* food.
Teeth – poor enamel, decay, abscesses.
Digestive upsets and diarrhoea, worse from *hot drinks.*
Irritant diarrhoea – sore anus and fissures.
Rheumatic complaints, worse from heat, better from motion. Numbness of limbs.
(Pulsatilla is heavier, softer, tired from exertion, chilled by cold water.)

Arsenicum Album (Group 5)
Highly-strung, nervy, finely-built, delicate-looking with fine skin and hair.
Chilly, like to be covered but want head cool, especially with congestive headaches. Cold, clammy sweat.
Scared, *frightened* of anything unusual, of the dark, being alone, going out alone. *Vivid* imagination. Night terrors.
Want to be comforted, consoled, somebody there.
Restless. Always doing something, going from one thing to another, or if nervous from one person to another.
Suddenly exhausted after activity, pale, wants to lie down, feels ill and frightened.
Tidy – hate mess – distressed out of all proportion.
Liable to catch cold.

Acute coryza, burning watery discharge, sneezing, tending to go rapidly into bronchitis, often with hoarseness between the cold and the chest symptoms.

Or, sudden acute tight *asthma* – terrified. Occurring 1–3 p.m. or a.m. Then frothy white sputum.

Very sensitive to cold, which leads to respiratory or gastric symptoms.

Digestive upset from exposure to cold, or following ice-cream and fruit.

Pains are eased by warmth, and they prefer warm drinks.

Acute diarrhoea may develop – sudden onset with collapse, restlessness, exhaustion after each frequent small stool, grey, cold and sweaty. In acute states a baby may only be able to move his head constantly back and forth.

Hyperaesthesia – sensitive to smell, touch, noise, excitement.

They will get sick, nervy or have nightmares.

If pushed at school, headaches periodical every 7 or 14 days, lasting a day or two and completely prostrated; intense congestive headache worse from noise, light or disturbance and, as already stated, better from cold air or cold cloth.

Chamomilla (Group 5)

The Chamomilla child has certain similarities to the Arsenicum child, but also some characteristic differences.

Hyperaesthesia, acute sensitivity to *noise*, *pain* and people; intense pain which puts them into a frenzy of rage – they resent it, demand to have it removed and will strike you.

Intense *restlessness*, wants to be carried about, passed from one person to another, jogged up and down. Yells if you stop, and pulls your hair. Never satisfied with anything he is doing, gets tired of it, throws it down.

More irritable and excitable at about 9 p.m.

Flushed when angry, with hot head and often *one cheek red*.

Teething – one of the great remedies for this; cross at night, tender inflamed gums, flush of one cheek, worse from hot application or hot room, better from *cold* application.

Acute colic – usually from anger, or after screaming; with wind and diarrhoea, green stools. Colic relieved by *hot* application (opposite for teething).

Hot children, hot head, hot burning feet, which they stick out of bed.

May scream till they go blue, or even have convulsions.

Otitis media: doesn't want to be touched, *very irritable*, yells with pain, again one-sided flush of face.

Cina (Vegetable, with santonin as its principal substance) **(Group 5)**

	Compare: **Chamomilla**
Obstinacy	Unstable
Circumscribed red patch on cheeks and pallor around mouth	One red cheek
Dislike of being handled or interference – *tender to touch*	Mental resentment

Steady passive motion soothes.
Sickness, but immediately after is hungry.
Nightmares and terrors if a late meal.

Diarrhoea – white watery stool – particularly white.	Green stool

Relief from pressure – lies on tummy with colic.
Chilly – sensitive to draughts.
Irregular twitching of face muscles after excitement.
Touchy – can't see a joke. (Older child.)
Hyperaesthesia of head and scalp – do *not* stroke. Jar aggravates.
Yawning. Acidosis.
Restless with digestive upset; meningeal irritation – rubbing head into pillow – may develop squint.
Irritation of nose – red, itchy, picking it (not necessarily worms).

Magnesia Carbonica (Group 5)

Sensitive, nervous type of child with lack of stamina, poor muscular power and soft flabby muscles. Any physical exertion tires them out. Easily startled by unexpected touch. Sensitive to the cold, but better in the open air, and upset by changes in the weather. Flush and sweat of the face after hot food or drink.

Headaches. Violent, neuralgic, pains tending to come on at night, with marked *sleeplessness*. The older child is mentally tired out at school. Adolescents are dead beat in the morning and difficult to get to school.
Desire for meat or meaty tastes.
Aversion to vegetables.
Intolerance to milk; sour vomiting and pale, pasty undigested stools, *white*, soft and like putty or eventually watery and excoriating. (Cina has white stools also.)
Tendency to *bronchitis* with enteritis – stringy, difficult sputum like Kali Bich.
Skin *dry*, scaly, copper-coloured eruption of the scalp.

Ignatia (Group 5)

This remedy is often thought of only for hysterical women, but it has a much wider application and can be useful in children who are highly strung, bright, sensitive and precocious. They do well at school, but if pushed they start to react with nervous headaches. The headache comes on later in the day and is relieved by heat.

Although clever, they blame themselves if they start to go to pieces, and become depressed and melancholy. In a confined place, they get nervous, distressed, choky and faint. Strained expression, tendency to grimace, twitch of eyelid or blinking.

Writing may become shaky when under stress. Up in the air or down in the dumps. Very *sensitive* to noise, cannot stand this while studying, blows up and then weepy, and then quite unable to concentrate or think. Scared if they get nervous – afraid of something going to happen, of taking initiative or going out alone.

Digestive upsets – sometimes upset by simplest foods and yet eats and digests most indigestible food. (Contradictions.)
Also inflamed throat, relieved by solid food pressing on it.
Cough, irritating, spasmodic – on and on, or acute laryngitis.
Rheumatic pains, better from firm pressure.

Zincum (Group 5)

A nervous, sensitive, excitable kind of child. The Ignatia child is very bright and quick, the Zinc child is slow in reacting, slow in grasping what you are saying, slow in answering, more docile and less unstable than Ignatia. Delayed development, especially delayed puberty.

Tired physically and mentally. When tired they get a persistent aching pain in the lower cervical region, with burning pain down the back.
Cramp in the hamstring muscles in bed.
Restless, twitchy, fidgety – restless feet.
Chilly, very sensitive to cold.
Inflamed eyes from the cold, with chronic blepharitis and intense photophobia.
Sensitive to *noise*, especially *talking*. When the child is working, talking drives them distracted.
Generalised skin eruption in childhood.
Acute hunger at 11 a.m.
Tendency to bolt their food.

Chapter 21

The Nosodes

THE BOWEL NOSODES

These remedies were developed originally by Dr Edward Bach and then by Dr John Paterson of Glasgow, a bacteriologist as well as a physician. He was assisted in this work by his wife Elizabeth, and both published papers in the *British Homoeopathic Journal.*

The remedies were originally derived from cultures of stools, and were prescribed on the basis of the percentages of organisms found in the stools of patients. Since the advent of antibiotics it has been found difficult to grow non-lactose fermenting organisms from stools, so the remedies are now used mainly on certain clinical indications, or on their association with related remedies. They should only be prescribed in chronic disease. It is usually recommended that a single dose should be given and not repeated for several months, using related remedies in the interval. They can also be used as a starting remedy, where the picture of symptoms is not sufficiently clear to select a single remedy, but where the nosode covers a likely group of remedies, e.g. Morgan Co. (or Compound).

The bowel nosodes are usually prescribed in the 30c potency.

Bacillus No. 7
Mental and physical fatigue.
Unfit for mental effort, leading to extreme physical exhaustion.
Flatulence, fullness after food.
Feeble urinary flow, loss of sexual function, premature senility.
Asthma, catarrh, sticky mucus.
Low blood pressure and myocardial weakness.
Rheumatic nodules, backache, cannot stand long, faints easily. Sensitive to cold.
Related remedies are Bromine, Iodine and particularly the Kali salts, especially Kali Carb.

Dysentery Co.

The keynote of this remedy is *nervous tension*, particularly anticipatory in character. The patient has a tense facial expression, not fearful but alert and ready to react. He is anxious, restless, fidgety, timid and uneasy amongst strangers; easily upset by criticism. Involuntary movements, tics or twitchings (like chorea) occur. There is instability of the capillary circulation, causing blushing, frontal headaches from excitement, and claustrophobia. The skin may be dry, scaly and with circinate lesions.

Its most marked sphere of action is in pyloric spasm, and where pyloric stenosis is spasmodic rather than mechanical (in which case surgical operation is often required). There is dilatation of the stomach, vomiting and a 1 a.m. aggravation time. Often valuable in duodenal ulcer, particularly when the pain and spasm follow anticipatory or nervous tension. In adults, cardiac disorders with mental tension and palpitation may be helped.

We see the close relationship between Dysentery Co. and Argentum Nit. and Arsenicum Alb. It is also related to Kalmia. Nux Vomica and Lyocopodium also follow it well in gastric disorders.

Gaertner (Bach)

This remedy is very valuable in malnutrition, either from lack of adequate diet or failure to metabolise, e.g. in steatorrhoea, coeliac disease or following gastric operations, and in some cases of colitis. Correction of diet, and vitamin and protein supplements are essential, but Gaertner helps the assimilation of these. It used to be of value in marasmic children, and may well have a place in underdeveloped countries and among refugees with inadequate diet. Emaciation in malignant disease and in the elderly is a further indication.

The children are hypersensitive to all impressions, physical and psychical, with fear of the dark and being alone. They have active brains, but poorly-nourished bodies and poor muscular development. They are restless – wandering about looking at things, but their attention is not held.

The remedies most closely associated with this nosode are Phosphorus, Silica and Mercurius.

Morgan Co. (Bach)

The keynote of this remedy is *congestion*. It is selective on skin and liver, in headaches with flushed face, aggravation from heat and raised blood pressure. The congestive features are seen in bronchopneumonia, where the indicated remedy fails to act even in the acute state, or to clear up a residual infection; in pelvic congestion and dysmenorrhoea, flushes of the menopause, circulatory disturbances of the limbs, blueness, chilblains, varicose veins, oedema and hot feet, etc.; and in skin ailments with heat and itch – eczema, red, raw with exudate, itching and bleeding. Hence the relationship to Sulphur with its hyperaemia of the surface circulation, Carbon with its deep internal venous stasis, and also to Graphites, Petroleum and Psorinum.

In the digestive sphere – congestion of the stomach lining and the liver with dirty mouth, indigestion and bilious vomiting. A great remedy in gallbladder conditions, constipation and piles.

These patients have a red, coarse, blotchy appearance, are often introspective, anxious about their health and irritable with a tendency to depression.

It can be helpful in the congestion around the joints in arthritis. There are two sub-types of this nosode – Morgan Pure, which is closest to Sulphur and particularly good in skin conditions, and Morgan Gaertner, which is like Lycopodium and helpful in cholecystitis and renal colic. It is often useful in hiatus hernia and diverticular disease.

Sometimes giving the nosode Morgan Co. in 30c potency, followed by Sulphur in 3x or 6x tablets twice daily, can help the acute itching in bad eczema or dermatitis.

Proteus

The keynote of this remedy is *suddenness* and *violence*, with nervous symptoms and spasm.

Violent temper in a child with kicking. Emotional hysteria such as one connects with Ignatia and Natrum Mur., and petit mal attacks of epilepsy.

The element of spasm in peripheral vessels makes it valuable in Raynaud's Syndrome, along with Secale, and in some cases of cramp. Migrainous headaches with blurred vision and Menière's syndrome may be helped.

In the skin we find herpetic eruptions with pain out of proportion to the lesion, and angioneurotic oedema.

In the digestive sphere the sudden onset is important, either haemorrhage or perforation, without any previous stomach symptoms but with a history of nervous strain building up. This slow build-up of strain in business and society with a sudden catastrophe is typical of Western countries today. Needless to say, the patient with severe haemorrhage or perforation may require transfusion or surgical intervention.

Related remedies are Ignatia, Natrum Mur., Apis, Cuprum.

Sycotic Co. (from non-lactose fermenting cocci of intestinal tract)
The keynote here is 'irritation', particularly in relation to mucous membranes. Hence its value in all catarrhal states of the respiratory tract, the bladder and the vagina, asthma, sinusitis, enuresis, chronic cystitis, vulvovaginitis, leucorrhoea, albuminuria, gastroenteritis. We also find it of value in warty growths, enlarged lymphoid tissue of tonsils and adenoids, glands, and the irritation of synovial linings in rheumatism; meningeal irritation, convulsions.

The patients are pale, sallow, flabby and soft, with long eyelashes (like Tuberculinum Bov.) and sweat of the head.

Stools are excoriating, loose and offensive, with urgent call to stool on rising.

Cough occurs about 2 a.m. and is worse from change of atmosphere, and symptoms generally are worse from damp.

There is fear, irritability and temper.

Related remedies are Thuja, Nitric Acid, Natrum Sulph. and Bacillinum.

NOSODES FROM DISEASED TISSUE

These are remedies prepared from diseased tissue or infected discharges. They are potentised and do not contain active organisms, and are therefore quite safe. There are two main groups. The first are used either in prophylaxis or, more commonly, as a follow-up to an acute infectious illness, having no real symptom picture or proving. The other group have a distinct symptomalogy on which to prescribe.

Group I
    Morbillinum – related to measles.
    Diphtherinum – related to diphtheria.
    Scarlatinum – related to scarlet fever.
    Parotidinum – related to mumps.
    Pertussin – related to whooping cough.
    Variolinum – related to smallpox.
    Influenzinum – related to influenza.

Recently added are:

    Rubella nosode.
    Glandular fever nosode.
    Brucella abortus nosode.
    Coxsackie nosode.

Also:

> Staphylococcin.
> Streptococcin.
> E. coli nosode.

These are all used where a patient has *never been well since* a particular infection or has persistent sepsis. They are not generally used during the acute illness, when the indicated remedy should be given.

Potencies of allergens are now available and are used in single occasional doses where indicated. For example: house dust or dust mite, pollens, grasses, dog hair, cat fur, horse hair, moulds.

Remedies potentised from drugs or metals may be used to antidote the side effects or allergic reactions of specific substances. For example:

> Penicillinum.
> Cortisone.
> Soap powder and detergents.
> Nickel.

Group II

This group contains nosodes which have a fuller drug picture, and which may be used either on the symptom picture or if there is a past or family history of that illness.

> Tuberculinum or Bacillinum.
> Medorrhinum (gonorrhoeal nosode).
> Syphilinum (Lueticum).
> Psorinum.
> Carcinosin.

Most of these are described in more detail in Section III.

REFERENCES

Paterson, John, 'The Bowel Nosodes', *Br. Hom.J.*, July 1950.
Paterson, Eliz., 'A Survey of the Nosodes', *Br. Hom.J.*, July 1960.

SECTION III

MATERIA MEDICA

This section contains the symptom pictures of some of the leading homoeopathic remedies. These are only summaries, and in order to learn the full picture of the remedy, and in particular its 'essence', it is necessary to study the remedy in several texts. The most useful are:

Introduction to the Principles and Practice of Homoeopathy, C. E. Wheeler and J. D. Kenyon.
Homoeopathic Drug Pictures, Margaret Tyler.
Leaders in Homoeopathic Therapeutics, E. B. Nash.
The Patient not the Cure, Margery Blackie.
Classical Homoeopathy, Margery Blackie.
Homoeopathy in Practice, Douglas Borland.
Lectures on Homoeopathic Materia Medica, J. T. Kent.
Studies of Homoeopathic Remedies, Douglas Gibson.

These texts describe each remedy in the totality of symptoms. They also explain the principal mental and emotional states, as well as types of individuals who most benefit from that particular remedy. This is the 'essence' of the remedy, the grasp of which is so vital in chronic prescribing.

Chapter 22

Fifty-five Common Remedies Described in Greater Detail

ALUMINA

This remedy is one of the great antipsorics, like Graphites and Sulphur. It is an antidote to lead.

Although experiments to assess the amount of aluminium absorbed by cooking in aluminium pans suggest that there is only a slight increase over the normal physiological levels, there do seem to be people who are sensitive to it, and who are made ill by eating food cooked in aluminium utensils.

Characteristically the Alumina patient has a pale, greyish metallic look, often dry, wrinkled and old-looking.

DRYNESS runs through its symptoms, in the skin, the respiratory and digestive tracts.

It is a remedy of paresis, ptosis of the eyelids (Causticum), intestinal paralysis (Plumbum), causing slowness in passing urine, constipation and weakness, mental and physical, with heaviness of the legs.

A chilly remedy, but with a liking for open air.

Mentals
Slowness of mind, of comprehension.
Resigned feeling that he will go insane. Deep despair.
Sense of being hurried. The delayed action in functioning mentally and physically makes her feel everything is passing too slowly (time passes too slowly). This leads to apprehension that she will not be able to finish a job, a fear that something bad will happen.
Depressive and suicidal – on seeing a knife wishes to kill herself (to kill others: Platina, Arsenicum, Mercury).
May be intellectual but dull in the morning; more alert by evening, with fear and apprehension.
Feeling of unreality (Medorrhinum).

Hypochondriacal men, with lassitude and indifference to work, irritable. The physical and mental slowing is gradual and hardly noticed by the patient. Very similar to the symptoms of Alzheimer's disease.

Eyes
The eyelids are inflamed, sticky, burning, dry, with the lashes falling out.

Respiratory
There is dryness of the mucous membranes of the nose and throat, with a stuffed-up nose; and headache from chronic catarrh, the headache often on the vertex, better from pressure, and accompanied sometimes by vertigo.

Dry hacking cough worse in the morning, with hoarseness especially in singers. (Argentum Met. has a similar hacking cough and hoarseness during the day.)

Gastrointestinal
A feeling of constriction in the lower oesophagus.

Loss of appetite, eructations, eats indigestible things.

Desires – fruit and vegetables.

Aversion – meat.

Aggravation from potatoes and irritating things like salt, vinegar, pepper, spirits and tobacco.

Constipation – No desire, no power to strain, even with a soft stool – excoriation of anus with soft stool.

Skin
The skin is rough and dry with eruptions which crack, itch and burn and are worse from the warmth of the bed.

APIS (From the sting of the honey bee)

This remedy mainly affects the skin and serous membranes, throat, kidneys, meninges, pericardium and joints.

It is characterised by BURNING, STINGING pains, with redness and marked swelling and OEDEMA. There is great SENSITIVITY to touch in all areas except the head (which is relieved by pressure), and there is general soreness leading to RESTLESSNESS (like Rhus Tox., but not relieved by motion).

HEAT in any form AGGRAVATES; hot room, hot bath, hot applications. Violent sudden onset.

Mentals

Conditions resulting from grief, fright, anger, jealousy, suppressed eruptions.

Tearful, depressed, anxious, constant weeping and whining.

May be irritable, suspicious, jealous.

As infections become more severe the patient is listless, apathetic, indifferent and eventually stuporous.

In meningitis there is muttering delirium with sudden piercing cries. All the mental symptoms are made worse by heat.

Head

Hot and congested with sudden, stabbing pains worse on movement and better from pressure (other symptoms worse from touch).

Eyes

Inflammatory conditions of eyes, iritis, keratitis, trachoma, with redness, oedema of lids, burning stinging pains relieved by cold.

Face

Red, burning and stinging; of value in erysipelas.

In kidney disease the face is pale and waxy.

Tongue

Fiery hot red, or dry and trembling.

Throat

Red, smooth swelling with oedematous uvula, burning stinging pain, again worse from heat and better from cold.

Absence of thirst, even in fever.

Respiratory
Violent dry spasmodic cough with soreness and sensitivity of the larynx.
Sensation of suffocation.

Gastrointestinal
Vomiting – distension, tightness, inflammation, burning heat worse from
touch.
Watery diarrhoea.

Genito-urinary
Nephritis with marked oedema, with restlessness, drowsiness and lack of
thirst. Aching pain in the region of the ovaries, especially right;
dysmenorrhoea. Worse from local heat.

Skin
Urticaria. Itching intolerable, swelling marked, stinging burning pain and
sensitivity to touch.

Limbs
Trembling, twitching and jerking of muscle groups.
Inflammation of synovial membranes of joints, swollen, shiny; sharp
stinging pains, sensitivity and marked effusion. Restless, worse from
heat.

ARGENTUM NITRICUM

HEAT aggravates – hates stuffy place.
Desires cold air, cold drinks, cold food.

Mentals

A remedy with many nervous symptoms, particularly the excitement of anticipation of events, causing diarrhoea. Fears to make a fool of himself in public.

Irrational, does strange or foolish things; troublesome thoughts which make him hurry – walks faster and faster.

Fear of death, of crowded enclosed places, church, high places. Feels he might jump down. Feels high buildings will fall on him.

Overworked, overtired, mental exhaustion and trembling.

Impulsive in love and anger.

Head

Headache worse from heat, but better from firm pressure. Brain feels exhausted.

Gastrointestinal

Desires *sweet*, especially sugar, which causes diarrhoea, and salt, strong-tasting foods.

Flatulence and distension marked.

Pains in abdomen, epigastric and spreading to the left.

Worse after eating, better from vomiting.

Vomiting and diarrhoea together (like Arsenicum Alb.).

Diarrhoea often greenish, like chopped spinach.

Tongue either smooth, red and sore, or pale, dry and flabby.

Ulcerations – mucous membranes, mouth, bladder, stomach with bleeding.

Other Symptoms

Eyes often affected; ulceration, purulent discharge.

Worse from heat, better from cold.

Sensation of a stick in the throat (like Hepar Sulph.), but relieved by cold.

Palpitation lying on the right side.

Worse before and during menses with dysmenorrhoea from excitement, and heavy bleeding.

Numbness of the arms at night – also hyperaesthesia.

ARNICA MONTANA

This remedy is mainly known for its action in INJURY and bruising, although it has wider indications.

It is a remedy to be thought of in any form of trauma, after surgical operations, following the trauma of a cerebral haemorrhage or a myocardial infarction, in rheumatism, gout and in the elderly.

Mentals

Irritable, morose, sad, does not want to be touched.

Forgetfulness, absentmindedness, hopelessness, indifference. Sudden horror of instant death – in cardiac disease. Dreadful dreams and imaginings – will relive the horrors of an accident.

Says he feels well – when seriously ill.

Cold nose.

Head burning hot with a cold body.

Great fear of *being touched* because of sensitiveness, e.g. gout.

Head

Cerebral haemorrhage – preceded by bursting headache.

Haemorrhages in the eye; easy bleeding; ecchymoses.

Respiratory

Whooping cough – painful cough, spasmodic with blood-stained sputum, bruised feeling with aggravation from touch. Child is cross and fretful.

Stitching pains in the chest like Bryonia, but worse from touch.

Gastrointestinal

Foul breath and taste in typhoid-like illnesses, with stupor and coma.

Offensive flatus, stool and eructations.

Other Symptoms

Restlessness because the *bed feels hard.* The soreness is relieved by change of position. (Rhus Tox. must move – uneasiness better from moving. Arsenicum Alb. is anxious, no relief even when moving.)

Sensation as if bruised or beaten all over.

General weakness and weariness – of value in the elderly.

Pains in the limbs and joints in rheumatism, sore as if bruised.

Effects of over-fatigue, physical or mental.

Can be applied locally for wasp sting – better in 1c potency – five to ten drops diluted in a pint of water. Too long application may cause dermatitis.

ARSENICUM ALBUM

These patients are always extremely fastidious in their appearance, dress and habits. This is noticeable in their house or garden.

RESTLESSNESS, BURNING, PROSTRATION, MIDNIGHT AGGRAVATION.

Extreme *chilliness*, cold hands, rigors and chills like ice water going through him, with thirst during the sweat, but not much during the heat.

Cold air aggravates, except for the head, which prefers air and cold.

Restlessness is a constant symptom, hurried, pours out his story.

Prostration *out of all proportion* when symptoms appear trivial.

Burnings in all parts, better from heat. Discharges are acrid and corrosive – nose, eyes, leucorrhoea, from ulcers.

Aggravation *midnight* and *1 a.m.*

Mentals

Deep-seated insecurity.

Anguish, anxiety for himself, about his health.

Perceives events from a personal point of view – 'What will this event mean for me?'

Sadness, despair, feels it is useless to take medicine as he is sure to die.

Fears to be alone at night.

Fastidious in dress and habits, obsessed by the need for order and cleanliness – this arises from anxiety and insecurity.

A feeling of being vulnerable and defenceless.

Sensitive to surroundings, touch, smell.

Covetous of other's possessions. Possessive of people, selfish, takes but does not give.

Headache

Congestive, throbbing, burning better from cold. Periodicity 7–14 days.

Respiratory

Asthma; must sit up, breathless on moving, sharp pain in the right upper lung.

Suffocative catarrh on lying down.

Sneezing from every change of weather.

Gastrointestinal

Vomiting and diarrhoea, acute stomach and bowel pains, food poisoning.

Thirst for small drinks, especially *warm*, but also ice cold in acute illness.

In chronic illness may be thirstless.

Genitals
Herpetic vesicles – burning little ulcers.

Skin
Fine, scaly, powdery skin or thick dry scales.
Severe sepsis.
Itch and inflammation burning, but better from heat.
Hair soft and beautifully kept.

Other Symptoms
Bleedings anywhere.
Oedema with thirst (Apis without thirst).
May help pain and restlessness in inoperable cancers.
May bring back old suppressed eruptions (e.g. eczema).

AURUM METALLICUM

The main characteristic of all Aurum salts is SUICIDAL DEPRESSION with want of self-confidence, alternating with hysteria and a kind of hysterical excitement and anger. They are restless and hurried mentally, but aggravated from physical hurry.

Desire for open air (except Aurum Sulph.). Better from cold and cool applications, yet icy cold hands and feet. Aggravations on waking (like Lachesis).

Mentals

Depression and loathing of life.

May be correct, just, fair, responsible, hard working, but cannot confess his innermost feelings or express emotions.

Sensitive to criticism, easily hurt, anger from contradiction.

Joyless, discontented with circumstances, quarrelsome.

Full of self-condemnation but critical of others.

Throws himself into his work in a pathological industriousness to escape emotional life.

Feelings of failure, that he does not deserve his status or wealth or life – hence suicidal.

Apprehensive fear, hypersensitive to noise, which makes her anxious, dread of men, fear of heart disease.

Terrifying dreams of death, thieves, falling from a height.

Eyes

Ulceration of cornea and inflammation of iris.

Ears

Noises in ears.

Respiratory

Catarrhs; ulceration of nose and offensive discharge, everything smells too strong – has a putrid smell from his own nose. Nose red and swollen. Metallic taste.

Stomach

Craving for alcohol and feels better for it (useful in alcoholics).

Skin

Deep ulceration of skin, and malignant skin lesions.
Induration of glands.

Rheumatic
Deep boring, tearing pains in bones and rheumatic joints, worse at night.

Other Symptoms
Serious heart conditions and chronic nephritis, with albumen and blood in urine. Sterility.
The Aurum state may come on after syphilis, and from loss of property or the fear of this.

Note the many similar symptoms to those in Syphilinum.

BARYTA CARBONICA

A remedy of children and old age.

CHILLINESS, sensitive to cold except PRESSING HEADACHE, which is better in the open air.

Emaciation, weakness. Pale, withered face.

ENLARGED GLANDS, particularly tonsillar but also generalised, chronic and indurated. Also mesenteric.

Degenerative conditions, cardiovascular, aneurysm, cerebral.

Prostatic hypertrophy.

Mentals

In child, slow learning to walk.

Slowness of maturing in adolescent and young adult.

Mental dwarfishness.

Loss of memory, mental weakness, confusion, loss of confidence. Aversion to strangers, shy child, timid. Irresolution – will make an excuse to avoid making a decision.

Premature old age – childlike behaviour in old person, or in an adult, suffering with deep emotional stress.

Want of clear consciousness in elderly – not clear in his intellect.

The *child* hides, easily frightened, imagines all sorts of strange things, cannot comprehend or memorise.

Sits and sits, lack of ability to think. Fear of something going to happen (Causticum). Whining, hatching up complaints and grievances.

Thinking of troubles makes them worse.

Ears

Noises, crackling when swallowing, associated with enlarged tonsils and glands.

Mouth and Throat

Dry mouth, bad taste, burning tongue. Weakness and paralysis of tongue in old people.

Throat – chronic suppuration, slow onset, granular-looking.

Blocking and gagging with solid food.

Spasm in the oesophagus when food goes down – in the elderly.

Respiratory

Coryza with swollen upper lips, thick yellow mucus, scabs and bleeding.

Weakness of voice, huskiness.

Dry suffocative cough. *Rattling in trachea*, aggravated by cold weather. Cannot expectorate. (Senega, Ammonium Carb., Baryta Mur.)

Heart
Palpitation worse lying on the left side, and worse thinking of it.

Gastrointestinal
Weakness of digestion, wind, hiccup and pain after food.
Constipation – lack of action, knotty stools, piles protrude.

Other Symptoms
Granular, sticky eyelids.
Dry eruption on the scalp in infants.
Gouty rheumatic pains, worse from cold.
Offensive perspiration of feet, causing soreness, ulceration.

BRYONIA

There are certain marked characteristics of this remedy. Intense AGGRAVATION from any MOVEMENT. This applies to headache, joint pains or pleurisy and, in the mental sphere, to any disturbance or exertion.

DRYNESS of serous or mucous membranes – dry mouth, dry intestinal mucosa with hard stools, dry cough and dry pleurisy. COLD, DRY, east WINDS aggravate and yet most Bryonia symptoms are worse in warm weather, warm room or getting overheated. There is a general relief from cold, and cold applications.

PRESSURE relieves – joint, headache, chest pain, except abdominal pains, which are worse from pressure.

Time aggravation at 9 p.m. or early morning, 3 a.m.

Mentals

Bad temper and irritability, dislikes being disturbed when acutely ill, will not talk if he can help it. When seriously ill with pneumonia or fever he will be still like a log, with dulled senses and intellect, resenting any interference or questioning.

Fits of anger, weak memory, delirium and dreams of his business or events of the day. A child keeps wanting something and does not know what. Despondent, anxious with fear of death and despair of recovery.

Insecure and lonely. Fear of poverty or financial disaster.

Headache

Severe dull throbbing pain with acute stabs over the eyes, relieved by hard pressure and cool applications, worse from movement and any exertion of mind or body.

Fever

Of value in influenza, typhoid and typhus. Marked *thirst* for large quantities at long intervals, profuse sour perspiration, dry lips and mouth with white or yellow tongue, as well as delirium and mental symptoms described above.

Respiratory

Laryngitis and tracheitis, with hoarseness and dry cough which is worse on entering a warm room and better from cool air. (Opposite of Phosphorus.)

Pleurisy with sharp, stitching pains in the chest, better from pressure or
  lying on the affected side (which prevents movement).
In pneumonia the patient looks heavy and dusky, with dry mouth, white
  tongue, thirst and perspiration, and is always better from cold air and
  cold applications.

Gastrointestinal
Pain and discomfort in the liver region, and even jaundice, epigastric pain,
  and in this instance worse from pressure.
Nausea, waterbrash and sour eructations, dirty yellow tongue and thirst
  for cold, although the stomach symptoms are really more relieved by
  warm fluid.
Stools dry and crumbling.
All alimentary symptoms are again worse from movement.

Rheumatism
Muscles, fibrous tissue and joint synovium affected, with pain, redness,
  heat and swelling from effusion, all aggravated by movement.
Pain is worse from moving. (Opposite of Rhus Tox.)
In acute rheumatism there is sour perspiration and irritability. Sometimes
  local heat will help, but more often cold applications relieve the pain.
Bryonia is often useful in acute conditions and is followed well by Natrum
  Mur. after the acute phase is over (e.g. in migraine).

CALCAREA CARBONICA (Impure calcium carbonate from
the middle layer of the oyster shell)

Calcarea patients are always susceptible to COLD, and dread the open air.
The least cold, and especially COLD DAMP weather, aggravates their
symptoms. Cold clammy feet, although they can burn when warm at night.
Hands are soft, moist, 'boneless' feeling and cold; chilblains frequent.
There is SLOWNESS, mentally and bodily, in movement, thought, learning
and growth. Physical and mental exertion exhausts.

Tendency to catch cold easily, to develop enlarged glands, polypi, leg
  ulcers and varicose veins.
Aggravation at 2–3 a.m.
The INFANT is fat, flabby and pale with a big head, slow closure of the
  fontanelles, and delayed dentition. Crusty eruption on the scalp.
  Chilliness with profuse perspiration of the head, soaking the pillow.
  Cough in teething children. Night terrors, sees things and wakes up
  screaming.
The ADULT Calcarea is also pale, flabby, phlegmatic, not necessarily fat
  but with a big head and scraggy neck.
Breathless, anaemic, chilly with tendency to palpitation.

Mentals
The child is lethargic, dull and just sits. She is clumsy, easily scared,
sensitive to criticism or being laughed at and feels useless. Also the night
terrors already mentioned.

  Older people are depressed, sluggish mentally, anxious about health
and the future, full of fears; that she will lose her reason, of getting a
cerebral haemorrhage, of what will happen, of the dark, of infectious
disease, of cancer, of death. Worries over others, over silly things,
sensitive to injustice done to others. Tears trickle silently down the face.
Peevish, obstinate, cannot think or remember – pauses before replying.
Fear that others will observe their confusion. May give up work, lean back
and let others look after them – parents may do this with their daughter,
although really quite able to do things for themselves.

Head
Vertigo and faint feelings. Headaches.

Eyes
Photophobia, sore in a cold wind; cataract.

Calcarea Carbonica

Respiratory

Chronic catarrh, nasal polypi, enlarged tonsils and adenoids.

Dry, irritating cough with pains in the larynx and chest, worse at night with wheezing and gasping.

Gastrointestinal

Desire for eggs. Eats indigestible things like chalk, coal and earth (children). Later in life they dislike meat, coffee and milk. Milk disagrees. They must have a good breakfast or else they get headaches.

Sour vomit, sour taste, dry white-coated tongue.

Distended abdomen. Constipation, but always feels better when constipated (laxatives upset).

Sour-smelling excoriating diarrhoea.

Genitals

Profuse and early menses.

Thick acrid leucorrhoea.

Limbs

Trembling, twitching, spasms. *Cramps* in the feet and calves on walking or in bed.

Weak ankles, pains in the long bones, wrists and between the scapulae. Back feels as if beaten.

Belladonna is the acute of Calcarea Carbonica. It would be used in an acute illness, and then be followed up by Calcarea. (Calcarea Carb. is also a chronic remedy related to Rhus Tox.)

CALCAREA PHOSPHORICA

One of the tissue salts, containing lime and phosphorus, and an essential for nutrition, growth and healing of bones.

In a small child there is slowness to develop and learn, slowness in closing of fontanelles, sunken abdomen, weakness of the neck and limbs and sweating. Colic in INFANTS after eating, and watery, green slimy hot, spluttering stools.

THE OLDER CHILD is thin, dark, but may be fair with blue eyes, growing with long legs, pains in the limbs. Cold limbs and face. Clammy skin, greasy (like suet pudding). The rheumatic pains are worse from cold wet weather, moving, in spring and autumn – with aching numbness and cramps. Neuralgic face pains better from heat, but worse on exertion and pressure. Muscular growing pains.

Mentals

The child is restless, going back and forth, reluctant to talk, tired with weak memory, discontented, peevish – always complaining that something is wrong (with school, etc.). Full of vague fears and dreads – especially in the evening. Fear of thunderstorms. Indisposition to work, cannot concentrate. Anxiety causes tummy upset and diarrhoea. Sympathetic, anxiety about others.

Headaches

In schoolgirls aggravated by mental effort, exposure to draughts, cold air, feeling of ice in the back of the neck. Amelioration of headache from bathing in cold water, worse from pressure, jar, exertion, tight hat.

Respiratory

Tickly cough – sputum yellow, offensive, worse in cold weather; head sweats, bronchospasm, better from lying down, worse on getting up. Pedunculated polyps. Glands in the neck. Chronic catarrh, better in a warm room, worse from cold.

Stomach

Good appetite. Desires tasty food, ham rind, kippers (but not so much salt as Phosphorus).
Upset by ice-cream, cold drinks.

Menses

Slow maturing and painful menstruation (cramping better with the flow).

CARBO VEGETABILIS (Wood charcoal, inert until triturated)

Hahnemann used only a 3c potency. Carbo Veg. affects mainly the vascular system, especially the venous circulation. Everything about the patient is SLUGGISH, lazy, full, distended, swollen and puffed. The hands are puffed, the veins are full, the body feels full and turgid, the head feels full, the limbs feel full so that the patient wants to put his feet up. There are varicose veins and ulceration with blackish or bluish patches, stagnation in the veins, poor tissues.

Generals
Burnings internally, in veins, head, skin, inflamed parts, stomach. But *icy coldness* of the nose, tongue, breath, knees and feet. Collapse with cold sweat, cold face and breath. Vital force nearly exhausted. Blueness of the face.

Mentals
The mental state is slow, sluggish, stupid, lazy. INDECISION, cannot concentrate. Great indifference, does not care if he lives or dies.

Head
Headaches mainly occipital, feeling of a weight, dislikes the pressure of a hat, worse on lying down.

Respiratory
Dyspnoea with expectoration, exhausting sweating and great coldness.
Acute violent spasmodic cough in paroxysms, with cold sweat and cold pinched face. Very useful in *whooping cough*.
In acute asthma and cardiac failure the patient wants to sit at the window or be *fanned*, even although he is cold and sweaty.

Gastrointestinal
One of the great *flatulent* remedies, full, distended with belching of wind, worse at night. Acid risings in the night. Offensive flatus. (Carbo Animalis is often better for relieving the flatulence after surgical operations.)
Desire for coffee, acid foods, sweet, salt. Loves to eat indigestible foods like puddings, pies, sauce and is averse to digestible food.
Offensive green diarrhoea.

A most valuable remedy for a collapsed patient, in a faint or even a heart attack, or post-operatively, where he is cold, pale, sweaty with a thready pulse, but wanting air.

CARCINOSIN (Nosode prepared from carcinomatous tissue)

(This drug picture is based largely on the observations of
Dr D. M. Foubister and Dr Dorothy Cooper.)

General Indications for Use

Where there is a family history of CANCER, tuberculosis, diabetes, pernicious anaemia.

Past history of whooping cough, pneumonia, glandular fever, amoebic dysentery or diphtheria, and the patient has never been well since that illness.

In chronic tonsillitis, sinusitis and headaches this remedy may be useful, and in the acute stage of glandular fever may be given three times daily for two days.

In acute respiratory infections where the patient at first seems to respond to the indicated homoeopathic remedy and then ceases to do so.

INSOMNIA.

Generals

Sensitive to extremes of either heat or cold.

Sea air either ameliorates or aggravates.

Aggravation undressing (cough, skin – Rumex).

Aggravation talking, laughing (cough – Phosphorus).

Better from short sleep.

Periodicity; worse from 1–6 p.m.

Alternation of symptoms from side to side (Lac Caninum).

The patient, especially a child, may have a café-au-lait complexion, blue sclerotics and tendency to tics and blushing.

Mentals

Mental inertia, tightness and constriction of the head, slow thinking, preoccupied and cannot concentrate.

Of value in mongols and psychotic patients with a suicidal tendency.

Fear prolonged, or prolonged unhappiness.

Anticipation – worry, anguish (exams, wife or child late home).

Fastidious – very precise, but occasionally the very opposite.

Obstinacy – strong sense of rhythm. They love dancing (Sepia).

Sensitive to music – makes them weep (Graphites).

Likes thunderstorm (Sepia).

Sympathetic to others (Phosphorus).

Sensitive to reprimand (Medorrhinum).

Where there is a history of strong parental domination or control from fear or sense of duty. The remedy Folliculinum is also strongly indicated in this situation, and may be given after Carcinosin.

Gastrointestinal
Desires salt, milk, eggs, meat, fat, fruit. Sometimes aversion to salt.
Constipation – with tightness and pain, worse 4–6 p.m., better from pressure, bending, hot drinks, sometimes with no desire (Opium).

Sleep
Disturbed, difficulty in falling asleep, with restlessness and shudders, excited dreams, overactive ideas. Lies awake most of the night or wakes 4 a.m. and cannot sleep again.
Insomnia in general.
Mental tiredness with headache (in students), better from even a short sleep.
Position in sleep – on the knees with chest down on pillow (also Calc. Phos., Lycopodium, Medorrhinum, Phosphorus, Sepia, Tub. Bov.) or on the back with arms above the head (Pulsatilla).

Skin
Eczema, especially front or back of chest.
Of use to prevent keloid formation, given before plastic surgery (Dr Paschero).
After reaction to vaccination.

Other Symptoms
Sensations of beating or throbbing.
Secretions tend to be thick and acrid.

CAUSTICUM (Potash preparation. See Hahnemann's instructions in Tyler.)

Sallow, sickly-looking, dark hair, dark eyes, dark mood. Paralysis, contractures, rheumatoid, warts.

After suppression of eruptions. Broken-down constitution.

Generals
Worse in cold dry winds, frost, causing paralysis, rheumatism.

Mentals
Hopeless, weepy, foreboding, apprehension, despair of recovery, fear something is going to happen, fear of dark, twilight.

Irritable, peevish and distrustful, but very sympathetic to suffering of others.

Ailments from grief, loss of sleep, anger. May sit silently, inattentive. Memory fails and mental effort leads to symptoms.

Can be angry, dictatorial, contradicting everything.

Vertigo
Worse on lying down in bed, worse on stooping, worse at menses; tendency to fall forwards or sideways. Sensation of space between brain and skull, better from warmth.

Headache
Pulsating or stitching, neuralgia of face.

Paralysis
Of single parts – *facial*, swallowing, voice – throat, eyelids, limbs with trembling (all like Gelsemium). Especially after exposure to very cold wind.

Eyes
Dry, stinging, itching; wants to dab eyelids.

Respiratory
Hoarseness worse in the morning (Phosphorus evening). Burning rawness. Loss of voice. Inability to raise sputum, partly raised and then slips back. Urine spurts on coughing. Cough relieved by cold water.

Stomach
Sits down hungry, but smell of food upsets (Arsenicum, Sepia, Cocculus).

Rectum
Paralysis – inactive, fills up, no desire – better standing up.

Genito-urinary
A most valuable remedy in cystitis – acute sensitiveness to cold. Great
   urgency with inability to pass urine, then later involuntary passage of
   urine without warning. Shooting pain in rectum when cannot pass urine.
Incontinence on coughing, sneezing or exertion.
Valuable following operation, when patient cannot pass urine.
Menstrual colic with tearing back pains better at night. Epilepsy with
   incontinence during irregular menses.

Warts
Hands, face, nose, eyes, large, bleed easily (Thuja, Dulcamara).

Rheumatic
Advanced with contractures of tendons, drawing pains, cannot get ease,
   restless at night. Worse in dry cold. Better from warmth and wet.
Slow progressive loss of muscle power.
Painful stiffness of neck and back on rising from a chair.
Drawing, tearing pains in thighs, legs, knees, feet worse in the open air
   and better in bed.

CHELIDONIUM MAJUS (Greater Celandine)

This remedy is best known for its effects in cases of jaundice or liver trouble and as a pneumonia remedy.

The most characteristic symptom is a fixed pain, either dull or sharp, under the lower inner angle of the RIGHT SCAPULA. This may occur in hepatitis or gallbladder disease or in cases of pneumonia.

Mentals
Forceful, opinionated people who tend to dominate others. Definite sense of what is right or wrong – will force his opinion on others.

Generals
Worse from cold, except headache and sinus.
Worse from change of weather.

Headache
Mainly in the forehead, supraorbital neuralgia and associated with biliousness or vomiting, brought on by heat and aggravated in a warm room or from warm applications.

Respiratory
In many ways resembles Bryonia in pneumonia. Right basal inflammation with stitching pleural pain, especially below the right scapula. The patient sits up perfectly still, as any movement causes pain, but unlike Bryonia, which likes pressure to the painful part, Chelidonium is worse from touch. Soon the patient will develop signs of jaundice or yellowness of the skin. Here there is relief from heat.

Gastrointestinal
Bitter taste in the mouth. Tongue thickly coated, yellow with imprints of teeth round the edge (Mercurius). Tendency to jaundice, stools whitish in colour, tenderness or stitching pain in the liver and gallbladder area, extending to the right scapula. It may relieve the pain in cholecystitis or gallstone colic.

Desire for hot drinks, hot milk or warm food.

Eating generally helps nausea, stomach pain or headache.

Other Symptoms
Rheumatic and neuralgic pains in the limbs.
Great weariness and drowsiness.

194

CHINA (Cinchona bark)

Chilly, sallow or jaundiced-looking patient. Pallor, weakness, nervous, sensitive to touch, motion, cold air; always catching colds, bowel and liver upsets. LOSS OF FLUIDS.

Debility
From loss of fluids, haemorrhage, sweating, diarrhoea, salivation, seminal emissions, purgatives. (Not the weakness of anaemia – Ferrum; not the nervous debility of Phosphoric Acid; not the weakness from loss of sleep and nursing, which indicate Cocculus; not the strain of over-exertion or overwork of Arnica; but the effects of loss of fluid.)

Hyperaesthesia
Extreme pain sensitivity, aggravated by *touch* or moving but better from *firm pressure*, e.g. in headache or abdominal distension.

Generals
Periodicity of symptoms – every other day.
Intermittent fevers – chill followed by fever, followed by sweat.
Thirst during the sweat, but not during the fever.
Persistent chilliness after influenza.
Very chilly.

Mentals
Emotional hyperaesthesia, oversensitive – dislike of company and a desire to be alone. Timid disposition, imagines people are being critical when they look at him. Considers himself ill-used, which leads to tempers, but not with the violence of Nux Vomica.

Gastrointestinal
Tongue flabby and coated, yellowish white.
Diarrhoea; painless, undigested, profuse watery stools with marked debility.
Flatulent distension *not* relieved by flatus or eructation, but better walking around.

Other Symptoms
Haemorrhages, venous in type, menorrhagia, post-partum.
Ringing in the ears. (China or China Sulph. of value in Menière's syndrome.

CIMICIFUGA (Actea Racemosa)

A remedy involving nerves (NEURALGIAS) and muscles (myalgias). Rheumatic, choreiform, spasmodic, hysterical and uterine, symptoms.

All improved from flow – diarrhoea or uterine, and yet symptoms are all worse during menstruation. Particularly a female remedy because of its relationship to uterine, menstrual and menopausal symptoms. Muscular rheumatism, pleurodynia, lumbago, torticollis.

Generals
Chilly, worse from damp and cold – rheumatism, neuralgias.
Cold forehead, pale, faint. Restlessness, jerkings, soreness and numbness.

Modalities
Better from warmth, open air, pressure, continued motion.
Worse from damp, cold, during menses.

Mentals
Fear of going crazy, imagines all sorts of strange appearances, that someone is going to kill her.
Incessant talking, changing from subject to subject (Lachesis).
Despondency – under a black cloud, overwhelming gloom. Wild, fearful expression, suspicion, fear of death.
Nervous, fidgety, excitable, irritable.

Head
Pains in the head as if the top would fly off. Shooting from occiput down the neck. Rheumatic pains in the neck, stiffness, as if pulled backwards.

Eyes
Shooting pains in the eyeballs, intense aching better from pressure and worse from motion.

Nose
Inhalation of cold air causes pain in head.

Respiratory
Short, tickly, dry, constant cough worse at night or on speaking.
Stitching pains in the chest, often intercostal.

Gastrointestinal

Nausea and vomiting, especially in females. Useful in pregnancy sickness if other symptoms agree.

Diaphragmatic pain – myalgia – pressing on the sternum and radiating to the oesophagus and pharynx, tingling in the throat extending to the shoulder and upper chest and to the arms and fingers. Worse after food and on walking, better from rest (possibly angina or hiatus hernia).

Genito-urinary

Pains in the uterine region, darting from side to side. Dysmenorrhoea, post-natal depression. Recommended in 1x potency during the last two months of pregnancy to help labour (Caulophyllum). Bearing-down sensations.

Menopause – sinking in stomach, pains in vertex, irritability.

Remember all symptoms worse *during the menses*.

Extremities

Rheumatic pains in cold damp weather, often on opposite sides, e.g. one shoulder and opposite knee. Rheumatoid arthritis pains worse at night and in wet weather, and also when associated with uterine problems.

CONIUM MACULATUM (Hemlock)

A deep-acting remedy. PARALYSIS, INDURATION, GLANDS. Hard infiltrated glands, breast lumps, induration of ulcers. Induration of testicles, impotency.

Mentals
Weakness of memory, progressive, mind becomes tired, cannot concentrate or stand any mental effort.
Complete indifference.
Unhappiness. Slowly-developing weakness of mind.
Will sit and mope in a corner.
Peevish, everything vexes him.
Any excitement brings on physical or mental distress.

Vertigo
When turning head. Worse lying as though bed turned in a circle, worse on moving eyes, better when eyes closed.
Sick headache on watching moving objects, cars.

Eyes
Weakness of eye muscles and lids, induration of lids.
Photophobia without inflammation – out of all proportion.

Gastrointestinal
Paralysis of oesophagus – food stops on the way down; feeling of pressure rising from stomach in nervous women.
Constipation – ineffectual urging, hard stool, paralysis of rectum, cannot expel contents.

Urinary
Urine flow will stop and start.

Other Symptoms
Cough dry, worse lying in bed.
Numbness with pains, or weakness. *Painless* complaints.
Weakness and increasing paralysis of muscles.
Stitching pains in head.
Tremblings, jerking and twitching.
Aching in legs from rheumatism or ulceration relieved by *letting legs hang down*.
Sweat *during* sleep – copious.

CUPRUM METALLICUM

Cramps, spasms, convulsions (cholera, whooping cough), twitchings. VIOLENCE OF SYMPTOMS. All symptoms RELIEVED BY COLD DRINK, (whoop spasm).
Dyspnoea, bluish lips, icy cold; violent spasmodic cough – also diarrhoea violent.
Cholera: Cuprum – convulsive.
Veratrum Alb. – cold sweat and vomiting.
Camphor – extreme coldness – dry.
Where inflammation and discharges cease and convulsions come on.

Mentals
Delirium, confused. Always likes to be occupied. Bored if idle.

Gastrointestinal
Metallic taste (Cocculus, Mercurius, Natrum Carb., Rhus Tox., Senega).
Eats *fast.* Desires cold food. Tendency to choke.

Limbs
Coldness of feet.
Cramps in the calves.

Related to the bowel nosode Proteus.

FERRUM METALLICUM

One of the four obesity remedies.

Palpitation, breathlessness, WEAKNESS EVEN AT REST.

Flushing of face on the least excitement, and yet cold.

CHILLY.

Pallid, waxy. ANAEMIA.

PAINS are worse at rest, better from slow gentle motion (like Pulsatilla); better from heat, worse on rapid motion.

Muscles flabby and relaxed. Prolapse: rectum, vagina, bladder.

Distension of blood vessels, plethora, varicose veins, and haemorrhages – nosebleeds.

Effects of fluid loss, like China.

Mentals

Sensitivity of nerves to pain. Restless, irritable, changeable in mood and impulsive.

Depression, anxiety, mental weariness. Upset by noise.

Head

Vertigo over water.

Congestive *headaches* better from pressure, worse on coughing.

Respiratory

Spasmodic cough, suffocative.

Gastrointestinal

Vomiting without much nausea – regurgitation of food.

Night vomiting. Diarrhoea on eating.

Aversion to meat, eggs, sour fruit.

Rheumatic

Pains – especially deltoid muscles, worse on motion, better slow moving, better from heat. More often on the right side.

GRAPHITES (Black lead)

Chilly, pale, obese women, although a valuable remedy in skin eruptions in men and women at all ages.

Sensitive also to a warm room, desire for open air.

Tendency to flush, and to nosebleeds.

SKIN ERUPTIONS often affect the bends of limbs, behind ears, scalp. There is oozing, thick, honey-like exudate.

Itch may occur all over without eruption, skin hot in night.

Discharges are offensive. Psoriasis also with scaling.

Cicatrices and scars can be softened by this remedy.

Mentals

Dull, lethargic, sad, despondent, lazy, weeps easily – especially at music – in a miserable way, timid, apprehensive. Irresolution and indecision.

Extreme activity of mind in the evening and first part of the night, keeping him awake.

Vertigo

On waking, looking up or rising from stooping.

Eyes

The eyes are frequently affected with marked photophobia, pustular inflammation, cysts and blepharitis with cracked, bleeding eyelids. (In Sulphur the lids are always red.)

Nose

Chronic nasal catarrh, with excoriation of nostrils, scabs and ulcers.

Face

Cracks at corners of mouth.

Cobweb sensation on the face.

Deafness – ear discharge. Hears better in a noise.

Gastrointestinal

Duodenal ulcer pain relieved by food and drink, relieved by hot food and warm milk, relieved by lying down.

Quite hungry, better from eating.

Averse to sweet, fish.

Constipation – knotty, lumpy stools with mucus or diarrhoea – undigested, foetid.

Extremities
Numbness in the forearms with cramps.
Nails brittle and deformed.

HEPAR SULPHURIS (Oyster shell and Flowers of Sulphur)

HYPERSENSITIVENESS (to touch, pain, cold air), OFFENSIVENESS, IRRITABILITY.

Generals

Aggravation from draught, putting his hand out of bed. (Silica is worse in wet cold weather, and better in warm, dry weather.)

Better in wet weather (warm wet). Aggravation from dry cold.

Glands, swellings, *suppuration* but painful, sensitive even to breath of air or touch.

Sweats sour, offensive night and day – without relief.

Discharges offensive. Eruptions moist, unhealthy, suppurating, sensitive.

Splinter-like pains (Argentum Nit., Kali Carb., Nitric Acid, Silica).

Mentals

Hypersensitive and touchy, irritable, *impetuous*, anger out of proportion, discontented, grumbles, resents coming to the doctor, sudden murderous impulses.

Intolerant to suffering, goes to pieces under stress, angry and nasty to husband or wife for no reason. Nervous excitement with hurry in speech or eating.

Eyes

Purulent eye discharge.

Ears

Ear discharge, mastoid – offensive and *sensitive.*

Respiratory

Suffocative cough, tightness (more than tickling) dry, deep cough – starts up wanting breath, worse on the *slightest draught*. (Spongia – hoarse, difficult drawing breath – narrow larynx.)

Sweats with cough, weeps with or before cough, wheezing rattling and asthmatic. (Like Natrum Sulph. but it is worse in damp weather.)

Stomach

Desires pickles and vinegar.

Mercurius, Hepar Sulph. and Silica, if following one another, should be prescribed in this order.

IGNATIA (Seeds of St Ignatius bean, containing strychnine)

The symptoms of Ignatia are PARADOXICAL, UNEXPECTED AND PERVERSE. They are also changeable.

If the patient is in the chilly stage of a fever and is cold, he wants to be uncovered.

When he is feverish and hot, he wants to be warm.

He is thirsty when cold and chilly, but not thirsty when feverish. The more he coughs, the more the irritation makes him cough.

When a part is inflamed, it is relieved by hard pressure.

When the throat is inflamed he gets relief from swallowing solids.

In stomach complaints it is the simple, unirritating foods which upset.

HYPERSENSITIVITY to pain.

Symptoms and pains are relieved by passing large quantities of urine.

Generals

Chilliness – complaints worse in cold weather and out of doors, better from sun, warmth, and clothing.

Rest relieves pains and movement worsens them; although hypersensitive to pain, it is relieved by hard pressure.

Pains tend to occur in circumscribed spots (Kali Bich.).

There are cramps, spasms and twitching of muscles, especially on the face.

Mentals

Although both Nux Vomica and Ignatia have strychnine in them, the Ignatia patient is seldom violent. She may be angry from contradiction, fright or grief, but feels that anger or crying is wrong. She is highly emotional, capricious, moody and changeable. Sensitive, refined woman with intuitive perception, quick to perceive, rapid in action. Hurt causes her to become harder.

Rapid alternation of moods – gaiety alternates rapidly with melancholy and tearfulness, but not so self-pitying as Pulsatilla. Symptoms often arise from sorrow at the loss of friends or from sympathy with the troubles of others. The effects of GRIEF on sensitive natures often calls for Ignatia – also mental anxiety and worry. These patients do not resent attempts at consolation, which occurs in Natrum Mur. or Sepia. Ignatia is a short-acting remedy in grief. It may need to be followed by Natrum Mur., where there are long-lasting effects and an inability to weep.

Headaches

Appear suddenly and are severe – aggravated by noise and light, and brought on by odours, especially tobacco. They are relieved by rest and warmth, by lying on the painful side, and sometimes even by stooping.
Pain like a nail being driven into the head (Thuja).
Headaches relieved by copious flow of urine (Gelsemium).

Eyes

Photophobia and flashes and flickerings of light, glittering zigzags with loss of central vision, but also conjunctivitis, lachrymation and blepharitis.

Respiratory

Dry, hacking, spasmodic cough, paroxysmal – the more he coughs, the more the irritation makes him cough. Whooping cough.
Sighing, unable to get a deep breath.

Gastrointestinal

Spasms in the throat, sensation of a lump when not swallowing, or better from swallowing solids.
Appetite capricious – either loss of appetite or craving for food. Cold food is preferred and there is dislike of alcohol, coffee, meat. Hiccough, vomiting and flatulence, often emotional in origin.

Genito-urinary

Copious urination which relieves headache.
Dysmenorrhoea – severe, cramping, labour-like pains with excessive flow and clotting, relieved by rest and by hard pressure (in the Ignatia type of woman).

Extremities

Violent sudden neuralgias, with cramps and spasms.
Sciatica on any movement, better from rest, hard pressure, heat.

Skin

Itching of the skin – often of value in the elderly with no evidence of skin eruption.

Natrum Mur. and Sepia follow well.

IODUM

INTOLERANCE OF HEAT. Restlessness.
INORDINATE HUNGER with EMACIATION – only feels well when eating.
ENLARGEMENT OF GLANDS everywhere except mammary, which wither.
Dark-haired, dark eyes, dark skin.

Mentals

Anxious and restless, must be on the move (like Arsenicum Alb., but this remedy is hot and Arsenicum Alb. is chilly).
Impulses to violence, especially if still – hence he walks about, hurries, and gets exhausted with weakness.

Respiratory

Excoriating catarrh, salivation.
Dry cough with stitches and burning, suffocative – all halogens (Bromine Chlorine and Iodine) have irritation of mucous membranes, with rawness, inflammation or croup.
Cough worse in warm room.

Gastrointestinal

Eructations, marked hunger better from eating.
Pains in the left hypochondrium and spleen.

Other Symptoms

Pains in joints at night in chronic arthritis.
Leucorrhoea yellow and corrosive.
Thyroid conditions, if other symptoms fit, with palpitation and feeling as if heart is squeezed (Lilium Tig.).

KALI BICHROMICUM

This remedy has particular characteristics and local indications rather than a constitutional picture. It affects mucous membranes and skin and is characterised by ulceration, stringiness, yellowness and pain in spots. Complaints generally worse in hot weather. Rheumatic pains wander from joint to joint and alternate with other symptoms, such as catarrh.

THICK ROPY DISCHARGES, particularly from the nose, throat and bronchial tubes, but also in gastritis and leucorrhoea.

ULCERATION of the nasal septum (seen in chrome workers), crusts, dryness, obstruction of the nose and tendency to bleed. Pains at the root of the nose and in the sinuses – may relieve where there is sinus pain and no discharge has come away.

ULCERATION of the throat and mouth – oedema of the uvula. Tongue is yellow and coated or glazed, red and cracked.

Mentals

A person set in his ways, proper, conscientious, rigid. Materialistic – enjoys home, family, car, food, traditional values and morals.

Does not like his deeper emotional world probed.

Weakness on a physical level and on emotional level – easily discouraged, feels isolated, gloomy and even sullen indifference.

Headaches

Blinding – sight returns as the headache intensifies, accompanied by dyspepsia. Violent headache aggravated by light, noise, better from warmth, pressure.

Stomach

Ulceration of stomach, punched-out, deep ulcers with emptiness, but easily filled (Lycopodium), wind and pain localised to a spot to the left of the xiphisternum. Vomiting sour and ropy mucus (sometimes in oesophageal diverticulum or hiatus hernia). Of use in the vomiting of drunkards.

Other Symptoms

Ulceration of the skin and legs; deep, punched-out. Bone pain. Pains occur in distinct *spots* on the head or in the epigastrium. They tend to appear and disappear suddenly. There is *yellowness* of vision, yellow discharges, yellow watery vomitus. Useful in measles where there are pustules on the cornea and pains extending from the throat to the ears, swollen salivary glands and catarrhal deafness.

KALI CARBONICUM

Pale, soft, flabby-looking people, with sweat on the slightest exertion. CHILLY, worse from cold, cold winds, cold applications (except piles). Puffiness of upper eyelids.

General aggravation of symptoms between 2–4 a.m.

Symptoms often RIGHT-SIDED.

STITCHING, CUTTING PAINS, WORSE at rest or on motion, from cold, pressure or lying on the affected side. (Bryonia better from rest, pressure.) These pains may affect the pleura, pericardium or joints, which are sensitive to pressure and touch. There is loss of elasticity and power in the ligaments and around the joints, causing slackness and weakness. Pains are often present in the right outer thigh between the hip and knee. WEAKNESS of the BACK with pain, in old people or for years after a disc lesion or childbearing.

Mentals

Drab, uninteresting people who tend to exaggerate symptoms, have a failure of will and inability to stand up to things, and hence keep returning frequently to the doctor. Strong sense of duty, inflexible, correct, proper, loves routine. Does not reveal her underlying emotions. Irritable, hypersensitive, on edge, startled by noise and may cry out when startled or with pains. A sudden noise catches her 'in the stomach'. Never at peace, tries to do several jobs at once and gets in a muddle. Fears to be alone, of the future, of dying or ghosts – imagination vivid.

Headaches

Congestive – over the right forehead and temple, severe and shooting, relieved by discharge of catarrh.

Respiratory

A remedy with much catarrh, frothy or stringy. Frequently catching colds. Sensation of a splinter in the throat (Nitric Acid, Hepar Sulph.) or of a lump. Of value in whooping cough and in asthma, particularly where there is 3 a.m. aggravation and the patient must sit up and lean forward.

Right lower lobe pneumonia, with hard cough and then tough muco-purulent sputum, and the characteristic *stitching pains*.

Heart

A potassium salt, and so we find a weak, irregular, intermittent pulse with low blood pressure.

Gastrointestinal
Desire for *sweets* or sugar – takes too much starch.
Flabby tongue, thickly coated at the base.
Dyspepsia in the elderly – full bloated sensation, with wind in the bowels.
 In pyloric ulcer the pain comes on two to three hours after meals, with
 vomiting of stringy mucus.
Feels worse from eating, especially hot food – distension after eating.
Colic usually associated with gallbladder. (Colocynth has colic related to
 the bowel.) If colic keeps recurring in spite of Colocynth, try Kali Carb.
 Burning piles are relieved by cold application.

Menses
Profuse.

KALI PHOSPHORICUM

Thin, pale, waxy skin, usually dark-haired with a tendency to flush after meals, with perspiration of the face.

Irritable, nervous, weak and PHYSICALLY EXHAUSTED.

Slight stoop on walking, with tendency to stagger due to weakness of the limbs.

Generals

Sensitive to cold, but warm weather also aggravates.

Worse in the early mornings (like Kali Carb.).

Worse from food, in the morning on rising, on exertion and before menses.

Mentals

Despondency, anxious, tiredness, lassitude, dislike of life (but not suicidal).

Irritability due to weakness, exasperation, inability to cope with their situation – they break down, weep and become exhausted, with tremor and fear – want to hold on to someone.

Shy, nervous of friends or strangers and suspicious of these, nervous away from home (fear of strange surroundings). In spite of this they may be obstinate.

Anxiety about the future, health, fear of crowds and of open spaces.

Sensitive to noise.

Emotional excitement causes trembling and exhaustion (bad news).

Head

Headaches especially in students – comes on in the night and on waking, improves when up and about, then worse in evening again.

Worse from cold, noise, mental effort, excitement.

Better from warmth, wrapping up, eating.

Scalp and hair sensitive to touch.

Cardiovascular

Weakness, palpitation, low blood pressure, anginal pain with numbness.

Gastrointestinal

Empty feeling but on eating feels full up, distended with flatulence; yet soon after feels hungry again. Nervous dyspeptics who nibble.

Desire for sweet biscuits, chocolate, sour things, vinegar and ice-cold water.

Aversion to bread, meat. Hunger at 5 a.m.

Inflamed tender gums which bleed, tongue flabby and yellowish.

Genito-urinary

Recurring acute cystitis with pain in the bladder region, incontinence in the elderly.

Scanty periods, excoriating leucorrhoea with ovarian pain.

Sleep

Violent dreams and nightmares.

Extremities and Back

Pain in the seventh cervical vertebra and dorsal spine when tired, with weakness in the back, worse from lying or sitting and better from gentle movement.

Numbness, tremor, pain on exertion.

Nerve degeneration (possibly of value in multiple sclerosis).

KALI SULPHURICUM

A cross between Sulphur and Pulsatilla.
Heavy, sluggish, high colour, slow movements, coarse skin.
Always tired – physical exhaustion, aversion to work.
Catches colds easily.
Generally worse from warmth, better in the open air.
Worse in the evening, but headache worse in morning.
Worse on exertion. Better moving slowly and gently.

Mentals
Depressed, lacks confidence – brain will not work.
Changeable – lively/depressed. Anxious about self, gloomy view of life.
Sensitive to noise.

Head
Congestive headache – feeling of heat, better from pressure and lying down. Mainly in the forehead and extending over the head, especially the right side. Giddiness.

Eyes
Itchy, gummed up, yellow crusts.

Nose
Intense irritation, ulceration, worse in hot room.

Ears
Chronic otitis media.

Respiratory
Cough better from cold air or cold drink.
Irritation in trachea, sputum yellow, difficult to raise.

Gastrointestinal
Yellowish tongue – insipid taste. Desire for sweet, sour, cold food.
Haemorrhoids with itch.

Sleep
During fever bad dreams of ghosts, death, murder.

Skin
Itch all over.

Rheumatic
Pains wander about, worse from heat, but feet and hands cold.

LACHESIS (The venom of the Surukuku or Bushmaster snake)

This remedy is characterised by BLUENESS, the blue bloated face in cardiac failure, blueness of veins, or ulcers which bleed and heal poorly. Petechiae and ecchymoses. Valuable in severe sepsis or pneumonia and especially at the menopause. There are several characteristic symptoms.

There is an AGGRAVATION of all symptoms AFTER SLEEP; pains or asthma may wake her; afraid to go to sleep because she feels so ill on waking. Marked SENSITIVITY to TOUCH, CONSTRICTION of tight things, especially round the neck, and to noise.

RELIEF from discharges, especially menstrual flow.

LEFT-SIDED symptoms – many of the Lachesis symptoms occur on the left side.

HEAT aggravates – faint in the heat, hot drinks aggravate, flushes marked.

Symptoms often OUT OF PROPORTION – sensations of choking, a lump or CONSTRICTION in the THROAT, are much more marked than the signs suggest. They are worse from touch, hot drinks, empty swallowing.

General aggravation of symptoms in the spring, and in mild, rainy, cloudy weather.

Mentals

Jealousy, suspicion (thinks people are trying to poison her).

Loquacity – talks constantly, going off on to other lines of thought, but sometimes may be slow of speech and taciturn.

Religious insanity – feels wicked and full of sin.

Thinks she is under superhuman control and may be commanded to do things. Disturbance of time sense. Sensitive to noise.

Headaches

Hammering or pulsating, often left-sided and worse from pressure and *after sleep*.

Cardiac

Palpitation with fainting, cramp-like pains, dyspnoea, and quick, irregular pulse. Anginal pain.

Gastrointestinal

Tongue trembles, is difficult to protrude, catches on the teeth. It is inflamed, swollen, painful – marked thirst.

Flatulence with intolerance of tight clothing, painful diarrhoea, spasms of the anus and large blue, bleeding piles.

Genitals

A wonderful remedy in the menopause, where periods are suppressed or have stopped, or where there are flushes and palpitation and feelings of choking. Increased sexual desire at the menopause. Dysmenorrhoea with pains in the *left ovary*.

LILIUM TIGRINUM

Usually fat and fair, poor colour. HOT, HURRIED, WORRIED – rather like a hot Sepia, but Sepia has marked indifference.

Mentals
Melancholy, silent, *depressed*, weepy.

Bad-tempered, a bit aggressive, angry. Exacting – things revolve round her. Feels she has something important to do, for which she alone is responsible, and no one else can do it, hence the hurry.

Full of fears – of going insane, of what happens after death, that she is suffering from a terrible disease.

Headache
With ocular disturbance and muddled feeling, from mental strain, worse at the menses.

Cardiac
Sensation as if the heart is '*grasped*' with palpitation – must bend double. (Opposite of Spigelia.)

Gastrointestinal
Desire for heat (unlike Sepia). Hungry even after a good meal.

Sensitive in the epigastrium, cannot stand a belt round waist.

Pressure in the rectum and *constant desire* for stool.

Genito-urinary
Pressure in the bladder with *constant desire* to urinate.

Sensation as if the whole *inside would fall out* through the vagina, not just the passive weight of Sepia, but a forcible pressure.

Cannot stand, must sit down.

This *intense pressing down* in vagina, bladder and rectum is characteristic of Lilium Tigrinum. (The bearing down of Belladonna is better from standing. The bearing down of Pulsatilla is worse from lying and better on moving.)

Uncontrollable sexual excitement with hurried feeling, worse before menses.

Menses heavy, clotting and irregular.

LYCOPODIUM CLAVATUM (Club moss)

This remedy comes from the spores of the club moss. These are inert until broken down by trituration, when an active ingredient is released. Lycopodium is indicated in patients who are pale, with a WORRIED FROWN, who look older than their years (prematurely grey). There is emaciation of the face and neck, with well-nourished body.

Often suited to intellectual people with responsibilities – lawyers, accountants, doctors, ministers.

Generals

Sensitive to *cold*, cold air, cold drinks, but headaches are worse from a warm atmosphere.

Symptoms are often *right-sided* or go from right to left.

Aggravation 4–8 p.m.

Worried frown on forehead and *movements of the alae nasi*, especially in pneumonia.

Mentals

Feels weak and inadequate – incapable of fulfilling his responsibilities. Constantly fighting against cowardice, moral, social and physical. Presents himself as capable, with extrovert friendliness and courage. Fear that others will find out about his inadequacy. Desire for sexual gratification without the responsibility of marriage – inadequacy reveals itself in marriage – may be impotent. Anxiety causes physical and emotional suffering – may try to escape responsibility by illness. Wants admiration and respect from others. May become a loner, spinster, celibate (Vithoulkas).

Anticipatory dread, fear of failure, aversion to undertaking new things, feeling of incompetence, and yet once he has started his speech or meeting he is capable and does well. Sensitive, emotional person with anxious worried thoughts, weeps on meeting a friend or receiving a gift, sometimes despondent and gloomy.

Fear of being alone, of crowds, dark, death, ghosts, and yet he does not want company, especially strangers. Wants someone in the house, but in the next room.

Eventually becomes domineering and imperious when ill, with taciturnity because he does not wish to talk. Then forgetful, making mistakes in words and writing.

Headaches

Worse from heat, warmth of bed, lying down.
Better from cold, cold air, better from eating.

Sore Throats
Most marked on the right side, or going from right to left, better from *warm* drinks.

Respiratory
Catarrhal affections of eyes.
Nose blocked, especially in infants, and then purulent discharge.
A remedy often indicated in pneumonia, especially on the right side, with a dry teasing cough, anxious look, flapping nose, and aggravation of symptoms or fever between 4–8 p.m.

Gastrointestinal
Frequently indicated in peptic ulcer, gastritis, liver and gallbladder complaints.
A very *flatulent* remedy (like China, Carbo Veg.); marked distension – must loosen her clothes, hungry and yet full up after a few mouthfuls. Wind in the bowel.
Desire for *sweet* food and *hot* drinks.
Aversion to meat, coffee. Upset by oysters.
Sour and acrid eructations.
Always worse from cold drinks and better from warm drinks.
Constipation without desire; also diarrhoea when other Lycopodium symptoms are present.

Urinary
Inactivity of the bladder with slow or feeble flow.
Deposits of red sand in the urine. Enuresis, and polyuria in the night.

Genitals
A remedy often indicated in impotency, especially if this follows overindulgence in sexual activities for some years previously.
Neuralgic pains in the right ovary, dryness of the vagina, delayed or suppressed menses.

Limbs
Restlessness and rheumatic pains relieved by motion and by the warmth of the bed. Worse in damp.
One foot hot, the other cold, numbness of the limbs.
Burning sensation between the scapulae.

MEDORRHINUM (Nosode made from urethral discharge containing gonococci. Being potentised it is safe, and does not actually contain these organisms)

A remedy of value in catarrhal conditions, ASTHMA, leucorrhoea and ARTHRITIS. It helps the general health and development of mongols. The person requiring this remedy tends to be plump, with wide nose, full lips and much hair, coarse and with bushy eyebrows. There is a tendency to have dandruff and tumours, sebaceous cysts, moles and warts. (The Sycotic type.) Several other characteristics are present. Symptoms often BETTER at the SEA. (Asthma, rheumatism.)

Generally WORSE during the DAY or 3–5 a.m. (Syphilinum worse at night.) DAMP weather relieves but cold weather aggravates. BURNING FEET. Worse before a storm, better lying on the stomach.

Mentals
Unstable, fitful symptoms which tend to be extreme in one direction or the opposite. Either *profusion* of discharges, temper, impulses, sexual indulgence or *inversion* with suppression, timidity, loss of physical and emotional power.
May be aggressive, forceful, wild with sexual thoughts or desires, or else weak, confused, forgetting words, dull.
Extremes – intense fondness for an animal or cruelty to it. Marked sensitivity to the beauty of flowers or completely uninterested in them (Vithoulkas).
Hypersensitive, dislikes being touched or having people around him.
Easily fatigued; aware of this and *hurries* in order to complete something before weariness and depression overtake him.
Physical *restlessness*, cannot keep still, fidgets.
Anxiety over the future, worries, depressed – even suicidal, selfish, fear of dying. (One of the *anticipatory* remedies.) Fear of insanity.
Difficulty expressing himself, loss of words, muddled, tendency to exaggerate.
Clairvoyance, sensation of *unreality* (as if outside of himself), time seems to pass slowly, and therefore he is disinclined to work or make any exertion.

Headache
Right frontal. Vertigo worse from stooping but better from lying down. (Conium is worse on lying.)

Respiratory
Catarrh, sinusitis, bronchitis.
Asthma relieved by lying in the *knee-elbow position*, with the face on the
   pillow (a strange symptom of great value in selecting this remedy).
   Remember also amelioration *at the sea.*

Gastrointestinal
Desires *salt*, sweet, sour, pickles, iced things.
Abdominal pains better from lying on the abdomen.
Green, irritating stools in babies.
Must *lean back* to pass a stool. Oozing from anus, with fishy odour.

Menses
Profuse, leucorrhoea which stains the clothing, sterility.

Urinary
Often of value in *enuresis*. Ammoniacal, scalding urine. Relief from
passing large quantities of urine.

Rheumatic
Arthritis better at the sea, worse during the day, with sensitive vertebrae
and lumbar stiffness. Pains in the heels. Damp weather relieves but cold
aggravates.

MERCURIUS SOLUBILIS (Black oxide of mercury)

Mercury is well known for its former use in the treatment of syphilis, and yet in fact there are many resemblances between the features of syphilis and the toxic effects of mercury. Possibly some of the action of the drug was homoeopathic in this disease.

The characteristic symptoms indicating Mercurius are: Sensitivity to CHANGES of temperature – aggravation from all forms of HEAT, especially the heat of the bed, but also from cold, open air or wet and damp. Seeks heat and is then aggravated by it.

Aggravation of symptoms at NIGHT.
Profuse SWEATING without relief.
Creeping chilliness in the early stages of a cold or fever.
Foulness of the mouth, with offensive breath. SALIVATION.
Lack of reactive power with inefficiency of function.

Mentals
Slow insidious weakness of reaction. In severe illness slow to answer or comprehend. Hurried and restless, but inefficient; may take a long time to do a simple task – not a productive type of hurry.

Impulsive – follows every random thought. Has impulses to strike, smash or kill, but controls these urges (Vithoulkas.).

Respiratory
Throat raw and smarting, with exudate or ulceration. The *tongue* is flabby, coated yellow or white, moist, and shows the imprint of the teeth round its edge.
Salivation with thirst and moist tongue, offensive breath.
The teeth are decayed or black, the gums spongy and bleeding, and toothache is frequent. Metallic taste.
Thick green or yellow discharge from the nose, with raw nostrils.
Otitis media in measles may be helped by Mercurius.
The *right* lower lobe of the lung is usually involved in pneumonia, and the patient feels *worse lying on the right side.*

Gastrointestinal
Desire for stimulants, preference for liquid rather than solid, and as already mentioned, thirst and *salivation.*
There is sensitivity in the liver region, worse from lying on the right side.

Acute colitis, and frequently indicated in dysentery or ulcerative colitis with slimy, bloody stools with colic and fainting and *marked tenesmus*, continuing after stool. (Can hardly leave the toilet, the urge is so marked – here Mercurius Corrosivus is usually better.)
May also be constipated with hard, knotty stools and mucus.

Genito-urinary
Nephritis, irritation at the end of the penis, nocturnal erections and increased desire, but great debility. Ulcers of the penis (syphilis).
Sweat of external genitalia.
Excessive periods, leucorrhoea profuse, excoriating and worse at night.

Skin
Eruptions of all kinds; papular, pustular, urticarial and chronic ulcers.

Other Symptoms
Inflammatory *rheumatism* with swelling of joints, worse from heat of the bed but also on uncovering. Bone pains worse at night.
Always the sweating and chilliness of Mercurius.
Tremor of the hands and tongue.
Great debility of body and mind.

NATRUM MURIATICUM

Pale, greasy skin, tendency to acne, emaciation in spite of eating, flushed on excitement.

These patients are reticent and nervous, and need to summon up courage to come to the doctor. Once there they are deliberate, covering their nervousness with a self-assured appearance, but showing tremor in their movements.

Generals

Worse from heat, better in the open air, but can be chilly. Worse at the *seaside*, but sometimes better with the sea air; aggravation from thunder. Worse about 10–11 a.m.

Intermittent fevers with chill but worse from heat. Thirst for cold during chill. Periodicity.

Desires – *salt*, fish. Thirsty.

Aversion – fat, bread, rich food, meat, coffee. Upset by milk.

Mentals

Vulnerable to emotional injury; any rejection, humiliation or grief is intolerable. Creates a wall to avoid being hurt. Sympathetic listener, but may appear cold or serious, not revealing her vulnerability. Guilt is a strong motivating factor.

Effects of grief or love affair; weepy feeling but cannot cry, yet weeps if consoled. Reticent, broods, harbours resentment, hates sympathy, but likes attention due to him. Not good at mixing. Sensitive to noise, music; startled easily.

Claustrophobia. Impatient. Poor sense of humour – tends to laugh when he should be solemn.

Instability (moods up and down), takes up with people and drops them. Nice to know but difficult to live with.

Sleep disturbed by unpleasant thoughts.

A child will suffer inside – from parental disharmony. If reprimanded will kick and scream – consolation makes her worse.

An adolescent will be withdrawn, sit on the sidelines, fantasize romantically – develop intense emotional attachments to people, keeping feelings to herself, but eventually breaking down in hysteria or sobbing.

Head

Headaches are hammering with zigzags in vision; may wake with headache. Sensitive to noise. Headaches midday to evening, especially in sun. Vision tends to give out on reading, eyes sore and tired, watery eyes in wind.

Respiratory
Coryza – thick white, but with dryness of mucous membranes, frequent colds, inflamed nose.

Gastrointestinal
Empty about 11 a.m. May eat much but remains thin.
Mapped tongue.
Constipation – dry, crumbling stool.

Genito-urinary
Menses delayed – feels worse at menses, not before it – backache.
Slow urination – cannot pass urine in presence of others.

Skin
Gluey, moist eruptions, itchy, exfoliating.
Herpes, crack centre of lower lip, painful spots on nose or chin, acne along hair margin.

Back
Vertebrae sensitive, yet relieved by lying on something hard.

A remedy often useful in nervous and emotional states, thyrotoxicosis, palpitation. Long-acting. Bryonia is the acute of Natrum Mur. – use Bryonia in the acute phase of headache and follow up with Natrum Mur. Apis and Ignatia are also related remedies.

NATRUM SULPHURICUM (Sodium sulphate, Glauber's Salts)

This remedy is most valuable in cases of asthma, rheumatism and diarrhoea, and after head injury.

It is a Sycotic remedy with warts, condylomata, catarrhal conditions and marked aggravation in DAMP and COLD, or near the sea. Symptoms are also worse in warm, wet weather (Lachesis, Carbo Veg., Silica). Sensitive to warm atmosphere, better in the open air.

Heat in the soles of feet and top of head. Coldness in the back.

Periodicity
Worse in the spring (Lachesis, Rhus Tox.).
Worse 4–5 a.m. – especially cough and asthma.
2–3 a.m. colic.
Diarrhoea *after* rising in the morning.

Mentals
Depressed, tearful, irritable in the morning, full of anxiety, sensitive to
    small noises; music makes her sad or annoys her. Cries in a quiet place.
Fear of the future, tired of life but does not really want to kill herself.
    (Aurum may commit suicide.)
Dislikes to speak or be spoken to. Mental exertion causes headache.

Headaches
Occipital, especially after *head injury*. May also have loss of memory,
    twitchings and even epilepsy after head injury.
Salivation with headache.
Noises in the ears.

Respiratory
Catarrhal – *greenish discharges* everywhere, nose, sputum, leucorrhoea.
Loose cough with pains and soreness of the chest – must hold his sides
    with his hands. Sputum green and salty. (Bryonia – dry cough.)
Feelings of oppression of the chest aggravated by damp.
Asthma worse from damp, at 4–5 a.m. and from sea air.
Left basal pneumonia with pains as above.

Gastrointestinal
Dragging and pains in the liver, bilious vomiting, nausea, eructations,
    flatulence and rumbling in the bowels. Colic 2–3 a.m.
Cannot digest starch, milk, potatoes.

Diarrhoea in the morning *after rising*. (Compare Sulphur – diarrhoea
   forces him out of bed.)
Feels better and more cheerful after stool.

Rheumatic
Rheumatic pains and rheumatoid arthritis, especially worse in damp and
cold. There is restlessness like Rhus Tox., but also aggravation from
motion, as in Bryonia.

Complementary to Arsenicum, Thuja.

NITRIC ACID

Tend to be dark-haired with brown eyes.
Great debility and lack of stamina of all the acids.
A CHILLY patient with profuse sweat of hands and feet.
Tendency to WARTS, ulceration, fissures, bleeding, offensiveness.
Indolent ulcers.
SPLINTER-like pains – in bone, throat, nose, anus.
General aggravation from WIND, thunder, WET.

Mentals

These patients are depressed, miserable, dissatisfied and despair of
recovery, anxious and yet *indifferent.* Irritable, intolerant of sympathy.
Bear grudges, do not forgive.
Suspicious, obstinate and restless. The irritability, especially in children, is
improved by travelling in a car or gentle vibration.
Sensitive to noise, pain, touch and jar.
Fear of death and cancer. (In some respects like Sepia, but Sepia loathes
fat and does not like salt.).

Sleep

Unrefreshing; irritable on waking in morning.

Headache

Fullness in the head, and a sensation of a tight bandage around the head –
sensitive to touch.

Respiratory

Nasal catarrh, acrid and excoriating the upper lip; nostrils ulcerated.
Cracks at the corners of the mouth. Buccal ulcers.
There is splinter-like pain in the throat on swallowing.
Offensive salivation like Mercurius.
Inflammation of the lungs.

Gastrointestinal

Dirty mouth, as described.
Desire for *fat* and *salt*, (like Sulphur), even although fat may disagree.
Orifices tend to be affected, mouth, nose, anus, vulva. Anal *fissures* and
piles – very painful, sharp and splinter-like pain lasting for hours after
stool, even a soft stool. (Nux Vomica pain is better after stool and the
pain in Mercurius lasts all the time.)

Genito-urinary
Inflammation and ulceration of the vulva; warty growths.
Urine with strong offensive smell like a horse's. The urine feels cold as it is
    passed.

NUX VOMICA

By nature the Nux person has a strong constitution, is ambitious, intelligent, quick, capable and competent with a strong sense of duty, efficient and hard-working. He will work all hours of the day and night. Competitive, loves responsibility, always believes he is right. Fiery temperament, offended at a harmless word, or malicious and IRRITABLE with anger and violence, and in extreme cases a desire to kill. Hates contradiction. Compulsive FASTIDIOUSNESS in pursuit of efficiency. Cannot sleep as business affairs crowd in upon him, troubled by many little details – may fall asleep after 3 a.m. and wake with a headache and bad taste. Worries over others, and may be sullen, quiet and averse to doing things. Uses stimulants, coffee, alcohol, drugs to achieve his aim. A remedy for indiscretion of eating, drinking, overwork and sex.

Generals
Chilly persons, worse in *dry* or windy weather, from draughts and yet dislikes stuffy atmosphere.
Burning heat with red face in fever, but cannot move or uncover without feeling chilly.
Sensitive to smells, noise, pain.
Spasms and convulsions made worse by the slightest touch on the head.

Headache
Dull headache in the morning after overeating or overdrinking, or when under stress.
Occipital headache in morning.
Headache associated with indigestion or liver upset.

Respiratory
Profuse coryza from one nostril, with obstruction.
Raw throat and larynx.
Early morning cough, violent and causing headache.

Gastrointestinal
Desire for tasty food, fat, rich food, which upsets.
Flush and fainting while eating, aggravation from meat.
Nausea with *much retching*, difficult to empty stomach.
Pregnancy sickness with sleeplessness. Liver congestion.
Dirty brown posterior half of tongue.
Distension and indigestion two to three hours after food.

Spasmodic constipation – with *ineffectual urging*, and sensation of incomplete stool with much straining and piles.

Colicky diarrhoea with nausea, hard lumps with watery stool, mucus and urging.

Also ineffectual urging to urinate.

Nux Vomica is an antidote to Sulphur.

OPIUM

Remember the opposite effects of overdose – first sensations of physical and mental happiness, stimulation and overexcitability, and then gradually stuporous. Opium is one of the few drugs which does NOT cause pain in its provings.

LOSS OF MORAL SENSE, lying and thieving – or, in children, lack of development of moral sense.

PAINLESSNESS – ulcers that are painless.

INACTIVITY and TORPOR – PARALYSIS – leading to the typical picture of the stroke patient.

Unconscious, stertorous respiration, jaw dropped, pupils contracted, face mottled, purple, hot with sweat, cheeks blowing out, and paralysis – no response.

INACTIVITY of bowel, symptomless constipation. (Prescribe in 6x potency twice daily for ten days.)

Inactivity of bladder – retention with full bladder.

AILMENTS from FRIGHT – where fear remains long after, paralysed with fear.

OPPOSITES. We can also see sleeplessness, anxiety, increased sensitivity to noise – can hear 'flies walking on the wall'. Delirium, eyes wide open, face red, puffed up. Vivid imagination, irritable, easily frightened.

Twitchings, jerkings, convulsions – in this situation he needs to be uncovered – wants cool air.

Bed feels too hot – wants to move to a cool place or be uncovered.

Failure of the patient to react to the indicated remedy would suggest the need for Opium.

PHOSPHORIC ACID

The most characteristic feature of this remedy is INDIFFERENCE and APATHY. WEAKNESS which starts in the mental sphere and then progresses to physical prostration, emaciation and debility.

It is indicated in people who are tired and apathetic from struggling with adverse circumstances, mental or physical, prolonged nursing of a relative – worn out. Children who are growing too fast and under strain at school. (China also has apathy and indifference, but the weakness is from loss of vital fluids.)

Generals
Cold, with tendency to cold sweats down the back or arms and hands, especially at night. Better from warmth, absolute quiet and being alone.

Mentals
Depression with listlessness, apathy and indifference. Ailments from care, grief, sorrow, disappointment, homesickness or unrequited love. In care and grief, Ignatia is the remedy of the sensitive, excited person with mood changes, but Phosphoric Acid has the apathy and indifference. In the effects of disappointment and resentment, Staphysagria is more intense and energetic, trembles and goes to pieces. In disappointed love, Natrum Mur. is more passionate, intense, weeping and hating sympathy, but not the dull apathy of Phosphoric Acid.

Lack of concentration, cannot collect his thoughts, slow to answer, talking exhausts him. Better from a short sleep (Phosphorus, Sepia).

Head
Crushing weight in the occiput and over the vertex, pressure in the temples. 'Brain fag'. Worse from being talked to.
Vertigo with ringing in ears.
Early greying of hair and falling of hair (Selenium, Natrum Mur.)

Respiratory
Weakness and feeling of pressure in the chest, behind the sternum, dry tickly cough, hoarseness. Takes colds easily which go to the chest. Salty expectoration.

Gastrointestinal
Craving for refreshing, juicy things; cold milk.
Copious, thin or watery, odourless, pale stools. In spite of the fact that this may be profuse, the patient is *not* prostrated by the diarrhoea but

actually feels better from it. This contrasts markedly with Podophyllum, which also has painless stool, which is yellow and very exhausting; the patient feels and looks ill.

Genito-urinary
Frequent, profuse milky urine.
Nightly emissions and impotence.

Extremities
Pains in the hip joints and long bones. Periosteal inflammation with burning pain, as if the bones were scraped with a knife.

PHOSPHORUS

The Phosphorus patient is usually tall and slim, either with dark hair, brown eyes and long eyelashes, and the pallor or pink and white complexion of those with a tendency to tuberculosis, or red-haired with freckles and a lively sensitive disposition. Constitution feeble with liability to catch colds and coughs, suffer from bowel or liver complaints and to bleed easily. Profuse sweats on exertion or in bed in the morning – sweat on the upper lip on exertion or mental effort. Bruises and bleeds easily, menses profuse, bright red.

Generals
Chilly patients.
Symptoms of the head and stomach are better from cold.
Symptoms of the chest and limbs are better from heat.
So we find the headaches are worse in heat and a warm room, and better from cold applications and from sleep.

Mentals
Indifference to loved ones, apathy, answers slowly, great sense of fatigue, disinclination to work. Unlike Sepia, Phosphorus patients crave sympathy, company, touch, stroking; need reassurance.
   Anxious, restless, full of *fears* – of thunderstorm, dark, death, that something will happen, of impending disease, cancer; hyperventilation, full of strange imaginings – vivid imagination in children. Artistic, extrovert, musical and often untidy. Attractive, sensitive people. Sleep helps – always better from even a short sleep.

Respiratory
Frequently indicated in chest infections. Hard, dry, tight cough which racks the patient; husky rough voice worse in the evening (Causticum in morning).
Cough worse lying on the left side, worse going from warm to cold air, from talking or laughing.
Sputum salty, bloody. Right lower lung often affected in pneumonia. Thirst for cold drinks.

Gastrointestinal
Stomach symptoms of vomiting, burning or bleeding are relieved by cold drinks, which are vomited after being warmed up in the stomach. Weak, empty sensation with desire to eat, and burning in the back between the

scapulae. Desire for *salt*, tasty food, sour and spicy, and craving for *ice cold drinks* and ice cream.

Chronic loose stools with profuse diarrhoea and loss of anal control. Sometimes bloody mucus and tenesmus, or long slim, hard, dry stools difficult to pass. (Of value in colitis.)

PHYTOLACCA DECANDRA (Poke weed)

This remedy is like Mercurius in many respects, especially in its throat and mouth symptoms.

It affects skin, throat, fibrous and osseous tissues, breasts. Symptoms worse at NIGHT, on COLD days, in cold damp weather, in a cold room, but also worse from the HEAT OF THE BED. Pains are SHOOTING – electric shocks worse on motion and at night, desire to move, but aggravation from motion.

Throat
Dry, rough fauces and pharynx, congested, *dark red* (Belladonna: bright red). Hot feeling like a ball of red hot iron. Swallowing difficult and painful – pain shoots to ears. Regurgitation from nostrils, inability to swallow even water.

Ulceration of mouth and throat. Irresistible inclination to bite teeth together.

Worse from cold in all things *except* the throat, which is *worse from hot*.

Mammary Gland
Mastitis – painful, inflamed, hot, unbearable, sore nipples with fissures.
Also indurated sore lumps, worse in cold damp. In nursing mothers, and also chronic mastitis, often troublesome during menses.
Of value also in cows with this condition.

Rheumatic
Rheumatic pains, burning, shooting worse at night and in damp weather. Inflammation of fibrous sheaths.
Pains fly like electric shocks, especially in deltoid attachment.
Shooting pain in right shoulder joint with stiffness and aching along the trapezius.
Tension and pressure in the parotid region – periarticular rheumatism.
Stiff neck – pain on the slightest movement (where Bryonia and Rhus Tox. fail).

PLATINA

Mentals

Lean, dark, sensitive, idealistic individual. Conflicting feelings of powerful sexual desire and an idealistic romanticism in her amorous affairs. This conflict leads to repeated disappointments in love. She wants her relationships to be fulfilling emotionally – this is often too much for a man to satisfy and she moves around from one to another. This may lead to nymphomania as well as to the ARROGANCE, haughtiness and CONTEMPT we associate with this remedy. She feels SUPERIOR and looks down on others – this loss of sense of proportion is also present in the physical sense too – things around her appear small. Often she desires to injure, physically or mentally, those she loves most. This may result in hysterical women from fright, shock, grief or prolonged excitement. The patient may feel deeply wounded and almost paranoid.

There are alternating extremes – hilarity and anger, wretchedness and excitement – following one another quite quickly.

Fear of death or that something will happen.

Headaches

Of gradual onset accompanied by numbness of the scalp and resulting from emotional causes, particularly sexual excitement or at the menstrual period.

Gastrointestinal

Flatulence, colic and constipation. The stool is clay-like and adherent with much straining. There is a sensation of retraction of the abdomen at the navel, like that occurring in Plumbum.

Genital

Symptoms in this region are often marked in this remedy. There is extreme sensitivity and hyperaesthesia of the genitalia. Increased sexual desire, sometimes with masturbation and nymphomania.

Pain over the left ovary, and heavy periods.

Other Symptoms

Pains generally come and go gradually. There is a feeling of numbness accompanying pain.

Sensation of constriction like a band round a limb.

Predominantly a female remedy, but not entirely so.

PLUMBUM (Lead)

This remedy has certain characteristic indications.

HYPERAESTHESIA, with extreme sensitivity to touch with LOSS OF POWER. This occurs in acute conditions. Where there is more chronic paralysis and weakness, sensation is also lost.

EMACIATION and MUSCLE WASTING.

PARALYSIS chiefly of the extensors, upper limb from the centre to the periphery (wrist drop). The paralysis is first local and then general, with difficulty in articulation or in passing urine, and coldness.

A remedy of value in progressive muscular atrophy (Hughes).

RETRACTION of parts. Violent abdominal pain with retraction of the abdomen and pain as if the umbilicus is pulled back to the spine. (Platina.)

Mentals

Indifference, depression, drowsiness and melancholy.

Although intelligent, the intellect is slowed – *slow* to remember, *slow* to answer, *slow* to react to pain (in chronic cases).

Hysterical, changeable, inclination to *deceive* – the patient may give a completely false impression of his home circumstances. Anxious sighing.

Encephalopathy with headache, visual disturbances and fits.

Gastrointestinal

Abdominal pain as described above, with retraction of the abdomen.

Obstructive symptoms with faintness and cold sweat. *Constipation with colic*. The colic is relieved by firm pressure.

Excessive thirst.

Blue line on the gums (poisoning).

Urinary

Chronic infections, with mucus and albuminuria. Paralysis of bladder.

Spasms

Neuralgic cramps, rectal spasm.

Feeling of a tight band round the leg. (Platina.)

PSORINUM (Seropurulent matter from scabies vesicle)

This remedy has similarities to Sulphur, but is characterised by marked chilliness and dislike of open air.

LACK OF VITAL REACTION – slowness of digestion, in passing stool or urine.

FOULNESS OF DISCHARGES – offensive breath, stools, leucorrhoea, eruptions.

Generals

Chilly. Generally worse in the open air or from draughts.

Skin symptoms often predominate. The skin is rough and dry, ichthyotic, with fissures, cracks and bleeding. Many types of eruption but usually *offensive*, oozing – pimples, boils, crusts, vesicles.

Eczema – very itchy and worse from warmth.

Scratches until raw. Worse at night. Better from cool air. This contrasts with the general aggravation from cold and open air.

Mentals

Depressed, hopeless, despair of recovery, thinks his business will fail.

Irritable, wants to be alone. Hates to be *washed*. Feelings of guilt, as if he has committed a great sin.

Headaches

Violent, throbbing, periodic, frontal – must cover the head (Silica).

Better after breakfast or eating. Must get up in the night to eat.

Eyes

Eyelids thickened and red.

Ears

Ears – eczema, scabs – also brownish, offensive pus.

Respiratory

Frequent colds with constantly running nose – very useful in hayfever, but also thick yellow discharge.

Dirty throat with mucus.

Asthma – cannot breathe in the open air, wants to go home and lie down. *Lies flat on the back*, with arms outspread. This is an unusual and valuable symptom.

Gastrointestinal

Hunger but nausea. Eructations like rotten eggs.

Stools watery, brown, *offensive*. Hastiness, urging (like Sulphur), flatulence (like Aloes), and difficulty in expelling soft stool (Alumina, China, Nux Moschata).

Other Peculiar Symptoms

Sick babies fret and worry and scream at night.

Patient often feels *unusually well* the day before or shortly prior to an attack (of asthma, diarrhoea or skin eruption).

During fever, patient is very hot and *sweating* profusely.

He also sweats with some relief after an acute illness, but is slow to recover.

Cannot bear limbs to touch one another (even fingers).

PULSATILLA (The pasque flower)

This remedy is often thought of as a remedy for women and girls, and so it is, but some men also fit the symptom picture. Frequently fair with blue eyes, tendency to be plump.

Generals
Pulsatilla is always *worse in a warm atmosphere*, and yet can be chilly in a warm room.

Better in *open air*, cold dry air (worse wet), better for *slow movement*; worse in the *evening*.

Changeable – in temperament, stools, rheumatic pains.

One-sided sweat of the face.

Mentals
Slow and phlegmatic, of a mild, yielding, tearful disposition, sorry for themselves. They laugh and cry easily. Like sympathy, but do not give it as easily as Phosphorus; they are also suspicious, jealous, irritable and peevish (not violent), touchy, feel slighted. Imagines certain foods are not good for her. Dwells on religious notions and thinks she has sinned. Malleable, attracted to dogmas or cults.

Fear of dark, alone, ghosts; of opposite sex; aversion to marriage.

The baby has a pitiful cry – wants caress. (Chamomilla has a snarling cry – wants spanking.)

Vertigo
With nausea, worse in warm room, using eyes, lying down.

Headaches
Worse in a hot room, using eyes; better in cool air, during motion.
Worse at menstrual period.

Ears
Otitis media or bland discharge.

Face
Eyes sore, red, itchy, styes. Crack in middle of lower lip.

Respiratory
Catarrh of all kinds, yellow or green, *bland*, better in open air, sinusitis, bad smell in the nose, with discharge, crusts, bleeding. Loss of taste and smell. Hayfever in a Pulsatilla patient. Cough dry in evening, loose in morning.

Gastrointestinal

Desires sweet, may like tasty foods which upset; fat and rich pastries disagree.

Sour vomiting and eructation – mouth foul in morning.

Absence of thirst, even with a dry mouth or during a fever. Likes ice-cream but it upsets if taken when patient is warm. Better from cold food and drink.

Bloated and distended – slow to digest.

Stools changeable, green; constipation with urging without stool.

Haemorrhoids worse lying still, better on gentle motion.

Genito-urinary

Frequent, scanty urine with urging. Lying on back causes desire to urinate. Involuntary urination from coughing, laughing, enuresis. Menses late or absent, scanty, intermittent and changeable, with colicky pain – suppressed after getting wet. Dragging-down sensations (like Sepia). Leucorrhoea may be bland like other Pulsatilla discharges but can be excoriating. Puffiness and swelling relieved by flow.

Strong sexual desire in male and female (in spite of mental fear of opposite sex).

Sleep

Cannot sleep till late on in night; dreams of cats; sleeps with hands over head.

Skin

Skin is hot, dislikes many clothes. Small brown patches of psoriasis or measles-like rash; also purplish spots (like Lachesis).

Limbs

Congestion of limbs, varicose veins, chilblains, hot feet in bed.

Rheumatic

Rheumatism moves about from joint to joint, always changeable but better cool.

Pains in limbs worse from hanging down (Vipera).

Often indicated in measles with the typical rash, sore eyes, photophobia, cough and catarrh and tendency to ear and chest complications.

Frequently useful in asthma or the recurring coughs of children.

Mumps, especially when male develops orchitis.

RHUS TOXICODENDRON (The great rheumatic remedy, also of
value in skin eruptions)

Rheumatic HEADACHE, feels sore in muscles, caused by draught or
DAMP, especially occiput, worse bending head backwards.

Rheumatic IRITIS from exposure to WET – pains shoot through the eyes to
the back of the head, worse at night. Orbital cellulitis.

Paralysis of eye muscles from exposure to cold and WET. Pain in maxillary
joints, cracking.

Stiffness and pain in neck and back, aching in SMALL of back. Strain of left
shoulder joint – pains in joint and arm, aching and numbness. Articular
inflammation.

Pains in wrists and hands.

Dull aching right sciatic nerve. Stiffness in knees and feet. Aching in legs,
unable to rest for a moment.

Paroxysmal pains from getting wet.

The pains of Rhus Tox. are worse on first moving but relieved by
continued movement. (Rhododendron pain is relieved immediately on
moving.)

Stiffness of part on FIRST MOVING.

Aggravation from draught, first movement, cold, wet, at rest.

Amelioration from heat and when warmed by exercise.

RESTLESSNESS. Must move the part. Pains worse AT NIGHT.

Numbness and twitching of extremities; traumatic paralysis.

Alternation with Bryonia as symptoms change.

FEVERS – with restlessness, delirium, suspicion of being poisoned.
(Influenza, paratyphoid.)

Dryness of the mouth with great thirst; red triangular tip of the tongue.
Desire for milk.

Effects of OVER-EXERTION of a group of muscles, or over-use of the
voice, which is initially hoarse and then improves with movement.

Mentals

Incapable of spontaneous warmth and expression, unable to relax, stiff on
the mental level also. Fear of being hurt.

Skin

Eruptions which are *vesicular* or pustular, or even erysipelatous.

Eczema of palms and fingers, blistering eruptions of the vulva, and
shingles. Herpes of the lips.

SEPIA

Sepia tends largely to be a female remedy, although occasionally we come across a male Sepia. She is thin, sallow with freckles or pigmentation and often a butterfly eruption across the nose and cheeks (like Rosacea). She has a dull, slow, stupid appearance, and yet can become vivacious, gay and sensitive, especially after exercise or dancing, which she loves. She complains of TIREDNESS, weakness and DRAGGING-DOWN sensations as if a prolapse may occur – she must sit down and cross her legs. She has low backache which is better from pressure and from active exercise.

Generals
Chilly with cold feet, but flushes easily and sweats in axillae, back and genital region. Faints on standing or kneeling and in a hot atmosphere. Usually better from sleep (Phosphorus).

Mentals
The characteristic of Sepia is a LOSS OF INTEREST and INDIFFERENCE, particularly to loved ones. She is irritable, weepy and cannot cope – wants to get away from things. She is averse to sympathy and yet dreads solitude, weeps on telling symptoms or at music, and is helped by a good cry. She is usually tidy but cannot be bothered; resents neighbours who try to help. Sensitive to noise; fear of incurable disease, insanity or poverty. Always better from active exertion or dancing, when she becomes alive.

Gastrointestinal
Desires – tasty, spicy food, vinegar. *Aversion* – fat, meat, milk. Empty feeling relieved by eating, but nausea at the smell of food or tobacco (pregnancy sickness). Constipation with fullness or ball in rectum – cannot expel stool and may have prolapse of rectum.

Head
Headache often associated with nausea and relieved by sleep, better from heat and pressure; worse from mental effort.

Genito-urinary
Irregularity of menses, too early or too late. Premenstrual tension, heavy period with only slight relief from flow. Burning leucorrhoea. May be of value in sterility. Dysmenorrhoea with poor flow. Involuntary urination, enuresis in first sleep.

Skin
Vesicular eruptions, herpes, warty lesions on the neck, and of course, the sallow appearance and tendency to butterfly eruption.

SILICA

A remedy often of value where there is SEPSIS, lack of reaction, failure to heal; for expulsion of splinters and pus in chronic lesions; induration of glands, especially parotids, fistulae. Tuberculosis.

Small, neat people with dull, lifeless hair; children have a big head and small body.

Generals
Chilly – pale 'dead hands' relieved by hot bathing.

Rough, cracked lips, fissures at the corners of the mouth, nails rough and yellow and poor quality.

Cold clammy feet and hands, profuse *sweats* of head and *feet* which are offensive.

Symptoms occur in cold damp weather.

Mentals
Lack of strength (not necessarily of 'guts'), exhausted by talking – therefore shy and dislikes talking to people. Submissive.

Resentful, overconscientious, but witty and good fun if brought out. Lack of confidence. *Dread of failure.*

Irritable, especially in the morning; child is cross and cries if spoken to. Anticipation upsets.

Headaches
Better from heat, wrapping up. Pain from occiput extending to right eye. Worse from cold, exertion, physical and mental.

Eyes
Inflammation of eyes, lashes fall out, crusting lids, blocked lachrymal duct.

Respiratory
Catarrh of ears, discharge offensive, yellow. Chronic recurring sore throats. Suffocative rattling cough, worse from cold or draught. Colds tend to settle in the chest.

Gastrointestinal
Likes cold food and drink; aversion to and upset by hot drinks or food, which make him sweat.

Milk upsets (Natrum Carb.). Recurring bilious vomit. Failure to assimilate (like Gaertner).

Constipation – lack of push – the stool slips back; offensive stools.

Sleep

Sleepless – wakes, thinks and worries and finally drops off, but feels better with even a short sleep.

Silica is the chronic of Pulsatilla.

STANNUM METALLICUM

Persons growing feeble over a long period; increasing WEAKNESS, cachexia, catarrhal conditions and neuralgia.

Sensitive to pain, increasing aversion to work, in business or at home; always tired.

Sallow complexion.

Great weariness, exhaustion on talking, weakness of the larynx and chest. The slightest exertion exhausts him.

Mentals
Despondent, discouraged, true despair – gives up the fight. Anxiety about the future. Distracted easily from one thing to another.

Neuralgia
Gradual onset, increasing, gradually diminishing. (Pulsatilla: gradual onset and sudden let up. Belladonna: sudden onset with intensity at once, ceases suddenly.) Usually in the morning, 5 a.m.

Sensitive
To cold, and every change of weather.

Headache
Every morning over one eye, especially left, spreading over forehead, increasing gradually and decreasing gradually, and often with vomiting.

Respiratory
Colds go to the chest – prone to tuberculosis.

Racking cough with retching; copious thick green, *sweetish* sputum. Coughs this up easily but more remains.

Weakness of the voice; hoarseness; talking makes him feel weak. Empty feeling in the chest, dyspnoea.

Rawness in the trachea. Paroxysms of cough, worse on talking, singing, laughing, lying on the side and from warm drink.

Gastrointestinal
Constipation; hard, dry stools, urging but cannot pass stool, which may be soft. Colic better doubling up.

Genital
In women a history of violent abdominal neuralgia, but once it goes she has a thick yellow-green leucorrhoea.

Menses early and profuse; feelings of prolapse.

STAPHYSAGRIA

This plant remedy has as its chief characteristic the mental picture. Almost all its complaints are a result of SUPPRESSED INDIGNATION, PENT-UP WRATH, and RESENTMENT. The patient becomes very angry but keeps it in, and then occasionally will let go and throw objects about. This anger can lead to headache, colic, rheumatic and joint pains. Takes offence easily. In adolescents with an unhappy love affair (like Natrum Mur.). As a result of this anger the patient trembles, loses his voice and cannot work or concentrate, becomes sleepless and develops headache. There is a great indifference and weakness of memory. Symptoms also develop as a result of sexual excesses or dwelling too much on sexual subjects. It is also of value in intense, energetic people with pride and envy (like Platina).

Vithoulkas comments that these people are often delicate, sensitive, highly-strung and considerate of others, and that in some cases they swallow their indignation without bitterness. Suppression of emotions, often in connection with romantic relationships. Reluctant to unburden themselves to the doctor, but if shown understanding will open up. They will accept grief with sweet resignation but still suffer from it – more romantic grief than death or financial disaster. An emotional wound never heals.

The other characteristic is SENSITIVITY, particularly to pain, with marked AGGRAVATION FROM TOUCH. Inflamed parts are very sensitive (like Hepar Sulph.), but there is also sensitivity to noise, tastes, odours. Decaying teeth in children are exquisitely tender.

It is indicated in the pain of INCISED WOUNDS or stretching operations (rectal or gynaecological).

Headache
Numb, dull pain in the occiput or forehead with pains pressing inwards and outwards, especially resulting from indignation, and aggravated by *touch*.

Eyes
A remedy for blepharitis, styes and nodosities or cysts of the eyelids. The eyes often appear sunken.

Gastrointestinal
Colic resulting from anger (like Colocynth and Chamomilla).
Diarrhoea and colic from eating or drinking.
Haemorrhoids very sensitive.

Genito-urinary

Irritable bladder with urging for days after pent-up anger.

A curious symptom of burning when *not* urinating, and less when actually passing urine. Cystitis after first intercourse (honeymoon cystitis due to stretching). Increased sexual desire in both sexes with impotence in the male, and shooting pain in the ovary and irregular menses in the female.

Condylomata and warts, especially round the anus or genitals.

Skin

Crusting, oozing, itching eruptions of the scalp, again very sensitive to touch.

Chronic induration of glands.

Rheumatic

Pains, arthritis and nodosities (arthritic or gouty), with stiffness and sense of fatigue in all the joints all worse from *touch*. Nightly bone pains. Pains particularly occurring as a result of anger, indignation or resentment, or accompanied by these, as often in cases of rheumatoid arthritis.

SULPHUR

This remedy is often thought of as a skin remedy, but it also covers many conditions in patients with characteristic sulphur general symptoms. It is Hahnemann's great antipsoric remedy.

BURNING, REDNESS, OFFENSIVENESS, DIRTINESS.

These patients often have a rough, dry, scaly skin, which breaks and suppurates. Skin lesions of all kinds, itchy, burning, worse from heat or bathing.

Boils, abscesses, severe acne, eczema, dermatitis, psoriasis.

BURNINGS in all organs, hands and feet worse from heat. PERIODICITY – every seven days.

REDNESS of orifices – lips, nose, anus, vulva. Eyelids red, crusty, itchy.

OFFENSIVE discharges which excoriate and burn. Congestion, varicose veins and ulcers.

Sulphur patients are HOT and aggravated by heat, but can feel cold and dislike wet and cold wet weather. Hot feet, which they put out of bed. Generally worse from STANDING, after SLEEP, after eating.

The typical Sulphur patient is lean, lank, stoop-shouldered, dirty and untidy (this latter may only be of one article of clothing, e.g. tie or jersey inside out), but some are stout, plethoric and cheerful. Children often look dirty and have coarse reddish hair – dislike bathing. (In spite of their mess, and offensive discharges and odour, they are very sensitive to bad odours – e.g. the smell of their own stools. They see beauty in ordinary things.)

Mentals

We often think of the Sulphur patient as a cheerful, friendly sociable, untidy person, but there are other less pleasant aspects to the personality. He may be introspective, selfish (thinking of himself), argumentative, with an aversion to work. He theorises, makes many plans and ideas, but cannot see them through (the ragged philosopher). Anxiety over salvation, feeling he will die, can become a religious fanatic, but loses his faith. Fear of losing his lucrative position, of the future, that he might become ill. Delusions that he is doomed, of misfortune, not loved by family or friends, being disgraced. Indifference to others and to his appearance, aversion to talking or being spoken to. This may develop either into impaired mental function, with poor concentration and absentmindedness, or into a more aggressive state with anger, agitation, fault-finding, hostility and suspicion, or impatient, hurried restlessness and even delusions of greatness. (Vithoulkas)

Headaches
Congestive like a band round the head, or pressure and heat on the vertex. Worse on stooping but better from warmth (unusual in Sulphur – the opposite of Arsenicum).
Dizziness, especially on standing, or rising in the morning.

Respiratory
Chronic *catarrh* with dirty nose and irritating discharge from nostrils, with redness.
Ears may discharge or are itchy, and deafness occurs from catarrh.
Inflammation at the base of the left lung. Sulphur will often help to clear up a residual consolidation or congestion in the lung after the acute symptoms have cleared up, but where there is failure of resolution.

Gastrointestinal
Desire for sweet, *fat*, butter, *stimulants*.
Empty, sinking feeling about an hour before lunch (11 a.m.).
Feels hungry, but on sitting down has a poor appetite, but marked *thirst*.
Flatulent distension with burning and colic.
Early morning *diarrhoea* which drives him out of bed, with burning stool, redness and excoriation round anus, and congested haemorrhoids.
Bad taste on waking, ulceration of the mouth, chronic sore throat which has a purplish appearance.

Genito-urinary
Urging and burning on urination, eruptions on genitals, burning leucorrhoea. In uterine haemorrhage or abortion, Sulphur is often needed to follow Aconite, Belladonna or Sabina as acute remedies.
Dysmenorrhoea in a Sulphur patient. *Hot flushes* at menopause (Lachesis, Sepia).

Rheumatic
Rheumatic conditions if general symptoms fit, especially if hands and feet burn.
Low back pain on rising, turning in bed.
Tendency to bedsores or corns and bunions on slight pressure.

Sleep

Restless and disturbed, wakes at 3 a.m. and cannot sleep again, dreams, hot in bed, throws off bedclothes.

General aggravation *at night.*

Other Useful Indications

Complementary to Aconite – its acute remedy.

Sulphur, Calcarea Carb. and Lycopodium follow each other well, in that order.

Measles with a marked purplish rash.

When symptoms occur as a result of suppression of eruptions.

When well-indicated remedies fail to act.

Where there are few symptoms to prescribe on.

SYPHILINUM (Lueticum)

A nosode prepared from a chancre.

Mention has been made in the text about Hahnemann's Miasms, syphilis being one. Patients may develop a wide variety of symptoms, either from a previous infection or if there is possibly a family history of syphilis. It is not a remedy to use in the active phase. As well as having a variety of symptoms and signs, there are a number of physical characteristics associated with this remedy.

Thin, dwarf-like persons with prominent forehead, retroussé nose, ears which tend to be small, or which stick out or are out of alignment; baldness, shining dry emaciated skin, drooping eyelids and shotty glands.

Of value where there are enlarged lymph glands, ulcers, contractures, abscesses, ovarian tumours.

Accident-prone, tendency to epilepsy, haemorrhage, hemiplegia.

Great weakness and exhaustion in the mornings.

AGGRAVATION of symptoms at NIGHT, at the SEA, in WINTER; better from motion and in mountainous country.

GRADUAL onset and disappearance of symptoms.

Mentals

Suicidal, depressed. Marked anxiety, fear about everything. Loss of self-confidence. Constantly checking things.

Constant inclination to *wash his hands*, because things he touches may be dirty.

Sleeplessness in the elderly.

Eyes

Ulcers in the cornea, keratitis.

Gastrointestinal

Craving for alcohol, cold food.

Salivation, cracked fissured tongue.

Prolapse of rectum and piles.

Genital

Acrid leucorrhoea, scanty menses.

Depression at the menopause.

Other Symptoms
Pains tend to run in a line – up or down. Patients are *not* sensitive to pain.
Tend to lie covered up if ill.

THUJA

This is Dr Compton Burnett's great remedy for the effects of vaccination, either where there has been a bad reaction or failure to react, or where the patient has never been well since.

Hahnemann's great remedy in Sycosis or following gonorrhoea. These patients look sickly, pale, waxy; are easily exhausted.

CHILLY, sensitive to DAMP, have CHRONIC CATARRH or WARTY GROWTHS. On exposure of the body to warm air there is shivering all over, warm air feels cold.

Profuse SWEAT on UNCOVERED parts; sweetish-smelling sweat.

Mentals

Reserved, suspicious, deceitful, manipulative, closed within himself – no deep communication with others. Irritable, quarrelsome, learns to control his base instincts and hence feels guilty. Tendency to act or talk hurriedly. Anxious about health or trifles. Weeps easily, especially at music. May progress to dullness, forgetfulness with mistakes in reading or writing. Speaks slowly as if at a loss for words. Prolonged thoughtfulness over decisions or replies.

Fixed ideas – as if the body was brittle and would break; as if the legs were made of wood; as if a live animal was in the abdomen. (Vithoulkas)

Headache

Accompanied by vertigo, neuralgias – sensation as if a nail were driven into the temple, or a tight band was round the head.
Headaches worse on waking or at bedtime.
Worse in heat, better in the open air.

Eyes

Conjunctivitis – especially gonorrhoeal. Nodules on eyelids.

Respiratory

Post-nasal catarrh and pharyngitis, affections of the mucous membranes, foul-smelling discharges, polyps.
Asthma worse in damp. May follow Arsenicum after the acute attack.

Gastrointestinal

Carious roots of teeth, pyorrhoea, gums swollen and inflamed.
Tongue red and painful; sweetish taste in the mouth.
A remedy to antidote excessive tea-drinking.

Eructations, nausea and wind.
Anal fissures, piles and warty growths, painful.

Genito-urinary
Pain anywhere causes frequency of micturition – pale, watery urine.
Sweat of the genitalia, offensive.
Gonorrhoea, warty-like excrescences, soft, sensitive and burning.
Periods early with severe left ovarian pain.
In the male, urethritis, prostatitis.

Skin
Scaly eruptions, pustular eruptions, herpes zoster, warts, cystic acne.
Effects of smallpox or vaccination.
Nails deformed.

Sleep
Wakes early and cannot sleep afterwards.
Dreams of falling from a height.

Other Symptoms
Rheumatism and arthritis, especially when related to gonorrhoea, leucorrhoea or pelvic symptoms.
Always worse in damp weather; foul-smelling sweats.

Thuja is often the chronic remedy related to Arsenicum, especially in asthma. Related to other Sycotic remedies – Natrum Sulph., Nitric Acid, Medorrhinum.

TUBERCULINUM BOVINUM (Prepared from tuberculous abscess or sputum)

This remedy should always be considered where there is a family history of TB, or a past history in the patient of tuberculous infection.

It is a remedy of intermittent fever – cases that relapse, or where a well-selected remedy acts and yet does not hold.

Recurring colds and coughs on the least exposure. Sharp pains in the left upper lung.

Loves wind and open air. Upset in a close atmosphere; sensitive to damp.

Periodicity 7, 14, 21, 28 days – periodic chronic headache.

DESIRE FOR CHANGE: house, travel, decoration, never satisfied in one place; cosmopolitan. Children may run away from home. Symptoms change – sudden onset, sudden cessation.

Mentals

Unpredictable moods.

Hopeless, aversion to mental work, anxiety in the evening, fear of dogs and especially cats.

Temper *tantrums* in children, destructive, disruptive, deep dissatisfaction.

Feels life is too short and hastens to make the most of it.

Gastrointestinal

Desires – salt, pork, fat, cold milk, alcohol; thirsty.

Emaciation while eating well – eats in the night, but also loss of appetite.

Constipation or chronic diarrhoea in the morning (Sulphur).

Genital

Menses early, profuse and long; also amenorrhoea, dysmenorrhoea.

Sexually hyperactive – tumultuous love affairs.

Limbs

Wandering pains in limbs and joints, stiff on first moving, better from continued motion (Rhus Tox.). Worse on standing.

Sleep

Dreams, waking 5 a.m., clammy sweats, especially at night.

BACILLINUM (Heath and Burnett's preparation from
TB lung, containing bacilli)

Deep-seated severe headache.
Cough with easy expectoration; sharp pain in the left scapula.
Pains in the glands of the neck.
Aching in teeth – sensitive to cold air.
Inflammatory conditions of the eyelids.
Restless, disturbed sleep.
Windy dyspepsia.

VERATRUM ALBUM (White hellebore)

This was one of Hahnemann's cholera remedies, along with Camphor and Cuprum.

Veratrum is characterised by COLLAPSE with prostration, COLDNESS, blueness and PROFUSE DISCHARGES. It also has marked mental symptoms.

Mentals

Ceaseless activity without purpose, hyperactive child.

A violent remedy in states of mental illness.

Delirium, destructive – wants to tear or destroy, tears at his clothes or pulls them off (like Hyoscyamus).

Religious frenzy, exhorts people to repent, despair of salvation.

Screams with obscene songs, lascivious or amorous behaviour. Fear of death or being damned.

Coldness

This is marked with shivering or rigors, *cold sweat* on the forehead.

Skin cold and blue, and yet there is *aggravation from heat.*

Copious Discharges

This may be vomit, diarrhoea, sweat, urine or salivation.

This loss of fluid causes collapse, fainting, rapid exhaustion and prostration, the skin becomes cold and blue, the face looks drawn and ill. Cramps may then develop (a typical cholera picture).

Fainting

May occur with less severe causes, from emotional stress or exertion.

The pulse is slow and weak and the blood pressure low.

It may be of value in cardiac cases.

Constipation may occur with large, hard stools, with colic, urging and again, cold sweat and faintness.

Pain

Neuralgias of all kinds, headaches and *dysmenorrhoea*, where there is prostration, cold sweats and vomiting. *Heat* always *aggravates* and the patient is restless.

ZINCUM

An antipsoric remedy indicated in feeble constitutions.

Nervous, excitable, sensitive to noises or talking, with tremblings, twitchings and jerking of muscles.

Incessant violent FIDGETING OF THE FEET or lower limbs.

Yet there is lack of vitality, 'brain fag', slowness of mind – must repeat the question before answering.

Anaemia.

Generals

Chilly – sensitive to cold.

Symptoms from failure of something to come out. Examples are: where a discharge or eruption has not appeared or has been suppressed by treatment; a child is restless, cries in sleep and rolls his head from side to side – once a rash emerges he is much improved; where the patient cannot expectorate but feels better when he does; where menstruation is of late onset, and the flow relieves (as in Lachesis).

Gastrointestinal

Hunger about 11–12 a.m. (Sulphur) – greedy.

Aggravation from wine or stimulants.

Sluggish bowel and bladder.

Rheumatic

Aching weariness in the nape of the neck, dorsal and lumbar spine worse on sitting, first rising, better from moving. (Rhus Tox. is often in the sacral region.)

Burning feeling along the spine.

HOMOEOPATHIC BOOKS FOR STUDY

Classical Homoeopathy, M. G. Blackie.
Dictionary of Practical Materia Medica, J. H. Clarke (3 volumes).
The Essentials of Homoeopathic Materia Medica, J. Jouanny.
The Essentials of Homoeopathic Therapeutics, J. Jouanny.
Everyday Homoeopathy, D. M. Gemmell.
The Handbook of Homoeopathy, Gerhard Koehler.
Homoeopathic Drug Pictures, M. L. Tyler.
Homoeopathic Prescribing, N. J. Pratt.
Homoeopathy, C. Ruthven Mitchell (An excellent historical book.)
Homoeopathy in Practice, D. M. Borland, edited by K. M. Priestman.
How to use the Repertory, G. I. Bidwell.
Introduction to the Principles and Practice of Homoeopathy, C. E. Wheeler and J. D. Kenyon.
Keynotes of Leading Remedies, M. C. Allen.
Leaders in Homoeopathic Therapeutics, E. B. Nash.
Lectures on Homoeopathic Materia Medica, J. T. Kent.
Lectures on Homoeopathic Philosophy, J. T. Kent.
Materia Medica of New Homoeopathic Remedies, O. A. Julian.
Materia Medica with Repertory, W. Boericke (Useful reference book.)
The Organon of the Rational System of Medicine, Samuel Hahnemann.
Organon of Medicine, Samuel Hahnemann, edited by J. Künzli, A. Naudé and P. Pendleton.
The Patient not the Cure, M. G. Blackie.
The Prescriber, J. H. Clarke.
Principles and Art of Cure by Homoeopathy, H. A. Roberts.
Repertory of Homoeopathic Materia Medica, J. T. Kent.
The Science of Homoeopathy, G. Vithoulkas.
Scientific Foundations of Homoeopathy, G. Resch and V. Guttmann.
Studies of Homoeopathic Remedies, D. M. Gibson, edited by M. E. Harling and B. Kaplan.

BOOKLETS AND SMALL BOOKS USEFUL FOR BEGINNERS

Elements of Homoeopathy, D. M. Gibson.
First Aid Homoeopathy, D. M. Gibson.
Homoeopathy – an Introductory Guide, A. C. G. Ross.
Homoeopathy, Born 1810, R. Livingston.
Essentials of Homoeopathic Prescribing, H. Fergie Woods.
Children's Types, D. M. Borland.
Influenza, D. M. Borland.
Pneumonias, D. M. Borland.
Digestive Drugs, D. M. Borland.
Homoeopathy for Mother and Infant, D. M. Borland.
Pointers to the Common Remedies, 1–9, M. L. Tyler.
    Especially useful are:
        1 – Colds, acute chest
        2 – Stomach, digestive
        5 – Infectious fevers

Available from: The British Homoeopathic Association, 27a Devonshire Street, London W1N 1RJ.

Introducing Homoeopathy into General Practice, R. A. F. Jack.
Comparative Value of Symptoms in the Selection of the Remedy, R. Gibson Miller.
Relationship of Remedies, R. Gibson Miller.
Study of Kent's Repertory, M. Tyler.
The Bowel Nosodes, John Paterson.

Available from: The Faculty of Homoeopathy, 2 Powis Place, Great Ormond Street, London WC1N 3HT.

GLOSSARY OF SPECIALISED TERMS

AGGRAVATION A temporary worsening of symptoms sometimes following the taking of a remedy, usually succeeded by a distinct improvement in the patient's condition.

CONSTITUTIONAL REMEDY A remedy on the basis of the temperament, character and general reactions of the patient (their constitutional type) as well as the local symptoms of disease.

DRUG PICTURE A summary of the symptoms, mental states and pathological changes that a substance is capable of causing (and treating) in human beings.

HOMOEOPATHY The system of medicine developed by Samuel Hahnemann invoking the principle that effective and non-toxic treatment may be given by using substances that can cause symptoms in the healthy similar to those the patient is suffering. This is summarised as 'similia similibus curentur' or 'let like be treated by like'. *Homoios* = like, *pathos* = suffering (Greek).

MATERIA MEDICA The homoeopathic pharmacopoeia; a list of remedies with their associated symptoms and uses.

MIASMS Conditions which may be acquired or inherited, and which have been postulated as the basic underlying cause of chronic and recurrent disease conditions. For example, Hahnemann considered all chronic disease to be manifestations of three miasms, syphilis, sycosis and psora, acting singly or in combination, and amenable to treatment by the appropriate remedies.

MODALITIES Those factors that qualify a particular symptom, e.g. pain worse from motion, better from local heat. Aggravating factors are often abbreviated to < and ameliorating factors to >. For example: pain < motion, > heat.

NOSODES Remedies derived from the products of disease (sputum, pus, etc.), diseased tissue or pathogenic organisms. The bowel nosodes are derived from culture of intestinal bacteria.

POLYCHRESTS Certain remedies which are very well known and which have a wide range of clinical application, often being prescribed on the patient's constitutional type.

POTENCY Most homoeopathic remedies are used in potency; in other words, the substances have been put through the process of serial dilution with succussion (or trituration if insoluble) at each stage of dilution. This is defined as potentisation and may be carried out with dilutions of one in ten (decimal scale), or one in a hundred (centesimal scale). A potency involving six dilutions on the decimal scale is written

6x (6DH in Continental Europe), while six dilutions on the centesimal scale is 6c or just 6 (6CH in Continental Europe).

Low potency: 1x up to 12x (6c).

High potency: 30c, 200c, 1M (1000c), 10M.

PROVING The testing of a substance on healthy volunteers (provers), who take repeated doses and record in detail any symptoms produced. (*Prüfen* – to test (German), from Latin *probare*.)

REPERTORY An index of drug symptoms, each heading or rubric listing those drugs known to cause the symptom. Often the remedies are printed in different type to denote the prominence of the symptom in provings and clinical experience; from black type, where the symptom comes through strongly, through italics to ordinary type. Hence 'black letter symptoms'.

SIMILLIMUM The single remedy that best fits the total symptom picture.

SPOT AND SPECIFIC PRESCRIBING This is a prescribing method, which, although based on the principle of similars, pays more attention to the local, particular signs of a disease, and less to the general response shown by the individual; e.g. Arnica, which is almost specific for bruising. Certain remedies also have organ specificities, and are prescribed on a pathological basis.

SUCCUSSION Violent shaking at each stage of dilution in the preparation of a potency. Traditionally the container is hit rhythmically against leather or the heel of the hand, but succussion is now usually mechanical.

TINCTURE Remedies in liquid form, normally with a mixture of alcohol and water as solvent. The remedy in its most concentrated form is known as the mother tincture, designated φ, and it is from this that the potencies are made by serial dilution and succussion.

TRITURATION Prolonged grinding with an inert base, usually lactose, in the preparation of a potency from an insoluble substance.

VITAL FORCE, OR DYNAMIS This term was used by Hahnemann to describe the innate recuperative power within the human body, which he envisaged could be stimulated by the homoeopathic potency. In disease, the vital force is disordered and the remedy helps to correct this.

Questions for Reflection and Discussion

PRINCIPLES AND PHILOSOPHY

What are the basic principles of homoeopathic prescribing?

What are the sources of homoeopathic remedies, and how are they prepared?

What is a potency? Can you indicate the commonly used potencies and when they are used?

List the main headings to be followed in taking a homoeopathic history in a chronic case.

What is the homoeopathic doctor's concept of chronic disease, its origins and progression, and what do we mean by 'directions of cure'?

What is meant by 'proving'? What other sources of information are used in compiling a homoeopathic materia medica?

It is often said that the second prescription is more difficult than the first. What would you ask at the second interview, and what possible alternatives are there for the next prescription?

What is meant by the prescribing of similars? Can you think of any instances of this principle in conventional medicine?

In what forms are homoeopathic remedies dispensed? How do you choose, and how would you give the remedy to the patient – in what dose, how often?

Describe your ideas of possible fields of research in homoeopathy, bearing in mind the difficulty of individual prescribing in the double-blind situation.

Write short notes on the following: a) General symptom. b) Particular symptom. c) Polychrest. d) Aggravation. e) Time modality.

What is meant by 'pathological' and 'organ' prescribing? Give five examples.

What is the importance of Past History and Family History in prescribing a homoeopathic remedy? Give illustrations.

A patient's personal reaction to environment and events (e.g. grief, fright, resentment) can often be altered by homoeopathic remedies. Name five remedies used in these circumstances, and what you would hope to achieve.

The appearance and behaviour of a patient is often helpful in selecting a remedy. Illustrate this with five common remedies.

MATERIA MEDICA

Describe the common accident and injury remedies and indications for their use.

Silica and Calcarea Carb. are both chilly remedies – compare and contrast their symptom pictures.

Give the indications for selecting three of the influenza remedies.

A child presents with a fever. What symptoms and signs would you look for in selecting a remedy in acute disease? Describe three acute remedies.

What features differentiate Sepia and Natrum Mur.?

How would you tackle a case of asthma from a homoeopathic point of view, both in the acute phase and in the longer term, illustrating with some remedy pictures?

Give details of six remedies of value in acute sore throats or laryngitis.

Compare and contrast Pulsatilla and Phosphorus.

A patient presents with symptoms of peptic ulcer. Describe how you would take the case history, with distinguishing modalities, illustrating your answer with remedies.

Describe a typical Lycopodium patient and his symptom complex.

In what ways does the picture of Nux Vomica differ from that of Lycopodium?

A patient presents with diarrhoea and colic. Describe some suitable remedies for this, with modalities.

Describe the symptom picture you associate with Phosphoric Acid.

Describe your approach to a child with eczema, and give details of the possible remedies you might prescribe.

Describe the symptom picture you associate with Sulphur and Graphites. Compare the similarities and differences.

What remedies would you think to prescribe in acute cystitis? Give details of the symptom pictures in these remedies.

Sepia and Lilium Tigrinum have some common similarities. What are these, and how do they also differ?

What do you know of the value of Causticum in respiratory and urinary complaints?

Three remedies often used in patients with leucorrhoea are Nitric Acid, Kreosotum and Hydrastis. Can you distinguish the leading indications?

Describe the modalities that would help you distinguish between four of the remedies for angina.

Describe the pictures suggesting Carbo Veg., Kali Carb. and Apis in cardiac failure.

What is the picture of Lachesis?

Describe and compare four remedies used in acute headache.

How would you approach a migraine case from a homoeopathic point of view?

Describe two remedies of value in the preventive treatment of migraine or chronic headaches.

Recurring sinusitis is a frequent problem in practice. What remedies might be used in the acute phase and also to reduce the catarrhal state? Give the symptoms in four remedies which would help you to prescribe in such a case.

Compare and contrast Rhus Tox., Bryonia and Causticum in the treatment of rheumatic disease.

Modalities are often very valuable in treating rheumatism or arthritis. List a few with their indicated remedies.

What symptoms do you associate with Ferrum Met. and Rhododendron in rheumatism?

Nash describes four restless and violent remedies. Can you list these and describe their chief features?

Aurum Met. and Natrum Sulph. are both remedies for depression. Describe their leading symptoms and indications.

Elderly patients can be helped by homeopathic remedies. What symptoms would suggest the use of Anacardium, Conium and Baryta Carb.?

Give a concise description of the types of children and their main presenting symptoms which would make you prescribe Calc. Carb., Silica and Phosphorus.

A child is brought with a history of recurring coughs, colds and wheezes. What questions would you ask the mother and what three remedies might help? Give their symptom pictures.

Compare the differences between two remedies used in children, characterised by burning – Sulphur and Arsenicum Alb.

What are the indications for the use of the bowel nosodes Morgan Co. and Sycotic Co.?

Describe the leading features of the two nosodes Medorrhinum and Syphilinum.

Appendix:
A Study of Kent's 'Repertory'

by Dr Margaret Tyler

With acknowledgements to Dr R. Gibson Miller, Sir John Weir
(from whose lectures this is mainly reproduced), and Dr Douglas Borland.
Reprinted by permission.

I hope it will be found helpful to have Dr Margaret Tyler's 'Study of
Kent's Repertory' printed here as an Appendix, in view of the valuable
insights it provides into the use of that centrally important work.

Dr Tyler published her Study in the June 1914 issue of 'The Homoeopathic World', and readers who have access to the original will see that I
have edited the literary style to bring it more into line with modern
usage. The homoeopathic content has in no way been changed.

H.W.B.

When one thinks of the bewilderment and despair of the uninitiated,
engaged in a first tussle with Kent's stupendous Repertory, one is
haunted by the story of the man of great authority from Ethiopia,
reading as he journeyed in his chariot, to whom a stranger joined himself
with the question, 'Understandest thou what thou readest?'; and the
prompt reply, 'How can I, except some man should guide me?'

'How can I, except some man should guide me?' There are mazes yet
that badly need the 'silken clue' . . . Kent's Repertory is such a maze.
With the thread in hand, you can penetrate with ease its deepest
recesses. But without the clue, you are lost.

It is questionable whether persons trained from the start in homoeopathy
can appreciate the difficulties of those who were never trained, but who
have had to pick out everything for themselves. They hardly realise the
difficulties faced by those who lack the clue to the scheme on which the
Repertory is compiled. Master the scheme and it is simplicity itself. You
can turn up, in a moment, what you want.

But – what do you want? . . . You have got to learn that too! For
without the knowledge of what you want – without the all-important

266

grading of symptoms, i.e. the realisation of their comparative value – life is too short, even when you have mastered its construction, to use the Repertory as your habitual guide in prescribing. And unless you do use it in this way, and commonly work out your cases, you will be unable to use it or trust it in emergencies.

For my part I can sympathise and understand, because I well remember my own difficulties. Until I first heard Dr Weir's lecture on the subject, in spite of having worked with quite a number of repertories for years, comparing them in the effort to deduce from them something simple and workable, I must say that I groped hopelessly in Kent, especially in the Pain sections. Rubric after rubric, at the interval of a few pages, seemed to have almost the same heading and yet a different list of remedies. The same ground seemed to be covered again and again, with a different result. How was I to choose the exact rubric and be sure of my remedy?

Remembering my own experiences and the illumination that came in one of the most important of an important series of lectures, I feel I must try to reproduce, in part anyway, the subject matter of that lecture, so that others too may grasp the idea and be made 'free' of the Repertory. Therefore to the uninitiated I offer this attempt at help, trusting that critics and experts may be able to point out any errors or fallacies.

Before considering where to look for what we want, let us pause to consider what we want to find. Knowing what we want to find will simplify our work and greatly limit our labours.

We go to the Repertory to discover the homoeopathic remedy. What *is* the homoeopathic remedy? The homoeopathic remedy is always that drug which, in its pathogenesis, exhibits the morbid symptoms of the actual patient we desire to cure.

The actual patient, to begin with. It is the symptoms of the patient – not necessarily the symptoms of the disease for which the patient consults us.

Hahnemann says the physician must realise that he is concerned not with diseases but with sick persons. In a patient we see a person who is suffering; an individual who deviates from the norm of the race and also from his own norm; a mortal out of tune to some extent with his environment, physical or mental, and therefore distressed.

If you are treating merely a case of some named disease, and attempt to hunt that disease through repertory and materia medica, you are very unlikely to discover the curative remedy. To begin with, remedies have seldom been pushed far enough to produce pathological lesions; and if your work is based on pathological changes, you are lost. Again, supposing many remedies had been pushed so far as to produce pneumonia, for instance, each would produce not only a pneumonia with symptoms peculiar to itself, but would also elicit symptoms peculiar to the individual provers. You would still need to individualise in order to cure. Pathologists know that drugs produce pneumonia or sciatica; what they do not know is that they produce a modified pneumonia or sciatica.

What you have to discover is the remedy needed by the patient himself; the remedy that corresponds to him, body and soul (and more especially soul). You need his individual remedy; the remedy for which the symptoms inherent in himself – not those dependent on his pathological lesions – cry out.

You may find many symptoms, all very pressing to the patient, which you may discard at once, since they will not help you in your search for the remedy. A patient with ankylosis is necessarily stiff. The stiffness appeals to him; on account of that stiffness he appeals to you, since it limits his movements and cripples his activities. But stiffness will not help you in your search for a remedy for that patient. It is a common and inevitable symptom in ankylosis, accounted for by the pathological changes.

Dyspnoea, with an enlarged thyroid partly impacted behind the clavicles, would be intensely distressing to the patient; but it would not be an important symptom, unless qualified, so far as repertory work was concerned. It would be a 'common' symptom, dependent on a mechanical cause. The remedy, unless it had been pushed to produce just such a lesion, would not need to have dyspnoea in black type. Dyspnoea, on the other hand, with nothing grossly mechanical to account for it, might lead to the consideration of certain remedies, especially if qualified by some modality such as 'Worse in wet weather – on waking – during sleep'. Or again, frequency of micturition, with a morbid growth impacted in the pelvis, would not help you in the choice of a remedy. It would be a symptom secondary to gross pathological change; not a symptom expressing the patient herself, but one dependent on mechanical pressure and promptly relieved by the removal of the tumour.

Symptoms dependent on a mechanical cause do not express the patient and are useless for homoeopathic prescribing. They may well lead to a more or less palliative remedy – palliative to the pressing distress – but have no value in the selection of the curative remedy.

Thus, before you open your repertory you can discard all the symptoms dependent on gross lesions, and so cut down a little on your work.

Which means – always examine your patient with care before you start with repertory. Be sure that the symptoms you take are peculiar to and characteristic of the patient himself, and not merely secondary to disease. But remember, you cannot eliminate symptoms dependent on a disease you have not diagnosed!

Besides pathological symptoms there are are common symptoms. These again will not help you at all, unless qualified. But they will cause you an immense amount of work if you choose to start on them.

Common symptoms are of two kinds. There are symptoms common to the disease, which are merely diagnostic and do not show how the patient reacts to the particular 'morbific agent', as Hahnemann puts it; and there are symptoms common to an enormous number of remedies, and therefore useless for the selection of one remedy – such as diarrhoea, vomiting, excessive sweating, headache. Common symptoms do not distinguish – and you need to distinguish – if you are to pick out the remedy.

Take the question of thirst; your patient has fever and is extremely thirsty. This is a doubly common symptom – thirst is common to very many remedies and to most fevers. You must have something more – something that distinguishes and qualifies to make the symptom useful to you; and yet the symptom is a general symptom, and as concerns the patient, urgent.

Enquire further and see if you cannot make it useful. Supposing you find that the thirst is at one particular time; or only during the cold stage, or before it; or that it is for large quantities, or small; or that there is thirstlessness during the period of high temperature only; or a raging thirst with no desire to drink. These things are peculiar to individual patients, and to fewer remedies, and are therefore distinctive. Underline them. You will be able to use them to find the remedy. You see how a common and useless symptom may be transformed into one of Kent's 'strange, rare and peculiar' – and therefore 'general' symptoms – because 'strange, rare and peculiar' must apply to the patient himself.

It is the same for all common symptoms, whether general to the patient or particular to his parts – diarrhoea, vomiting, localised pain, headache – the very ailments for which he comes to you for help. See what long rubrics there are, with almost every remedy in them! Never start on these. They are useless unless you can get something that qualifies or distinguishes, that is peculiar to this particular patient with diarrhoea or headache. If so, a common symptom that is qualified may help you.

But if we may not take the ailments complained of by the patient, nor the urgent and distressing symptoms dependent on a lesion, what are we to take? What are the symptoms that *do* denote the patient and on which we may start? And how are symptoms to be graded according to their relative importance?

Kent (following Hahnemann closely in this, as in all things) is most definite as to the symptoms of first grade – those of supreme importance to the case and expressing most absolutely the patient. These are the mental symptoms. If they are marked, they dominate the case.

You may find that a patient is intensely jealous, or suspicious, or tearful, or indifferent to loved ones, or reserved and intolerant of sympathy and consolation. In sickness these things come out. Often in sickness the very nature seems to change. The rash and reckless become timid for themselves and others; the good-tempered become snappy; the irritable and restless become patient. If a mental trait is marked, and especially if it denotes change from the patient's norm, it is of great importance to the case. It must also be in the same type in the rubric as in the patient, which means that only remedies in the higher types are likely to fit the case. If the symptom is not very marked, beware how you use it to eliminate remedies; if the rubric is very small, take it, but also take with it a larger rubric that more or less includes the trait. Do not risk missing your remedy for an ill-marked mental or a very small rubric. But if it is very marked, you know that the remedy you are seeking must be among the remedies in that rubric, so here again you may be able to limit your work.

Kent says, 'When you have taken a case on paper you must settle upon the symptoms that cannot be omitted in each individual.' Such a marked mental – mentals being of the highest grade – would be one of the symptoms that you cannot omit for this individual; your remedy must be here. You can therefore use it as an eliminating symptom, to compare with all the subsequent rubrics you consult; from this you can often discard the remedies that do not appear in this first essential list. With this strong eliminating symptom, straight from 'the heart of the patient's heart', you can go through the rubrics of the patient's symptoms in their order. That is, mentals first, then generals, then particulars with modalities, taking from each list only the remedies that appear in this first rubric (insane jealousy, or whatever it be), but taking all these jealous remedies from every subsequent list. In this way you can work rapidly down, till you are satisfied that you have found the remedy that fits the patient as a whole.

To eliminate with safety, you must take symptoms seriously, not lightly. You must be absolutely sure that your symptoms are real and marked; that they do actually express the patient. You will have to ask many questions to elicit a few telling symptoms, and you must be sure that you and your patient mean the same thing. There are many pitfalls.

Even the mental symptoms are graded. Of highest rank are those that relate to the will, with loves and hates, suspicions and fears. She hates her child – is jealous – fear of disease – of solitude.

The second grade are those that affect the understanding, with delusions, delirium, loss of the sense of proportion, exaltation of trifles, delusions of grandeur or persecution. Of third and lowest mental grade are the ones that relate to memory.

Then as Kent puts it, the 'strange, rare and peculiar symptoms are therefore among the highest generals; because strange, rare and peculiar must apply to the patient himself.' These take a high place in the search for the remedy, albeit a place depending on their grade, for a peculiar mental would rank higher than a mere peculiar local symptom. Many of them are indicative of one or two remedies only. Put them high in your list but use them with care. As Kent says, 'The great trouble with keynotes is that they are misused. The keynotes are often characteristic symptoms; but if the keynotes are taken as final, and the generals do not conform, then will come the failures.' Wiping out a symptom, and curing a patient, are not synonymous.

A remedy in its provings can only evoke in each case what was there already, latent in the prover – just as disease brings out weak points – and therefore does not affect any two patients in exactly the same way. It requires many provers of different types and different defective resistances to bring out the whole picture of a remedy pathogenesis. If more remedies had been more extensively proved, many more 'rare, peculiar and distinctive' symptoms would probably have seen the light of day. A patient's own individual remedy, prescribed on mental and general symptoms, will often eliminate peculiar symptoms which it has never been recorded as having evoked, and which are the striking keynotes of some other remedy. Beware therefore how you use rare and peculiar symptoms as eliminating symptoms, if they have only one or two remedies to their credit. It is easy to do this, but often fatal. They may put you straight on to your remedy (if the rest of the case fits). They may also put you straight off it. You dare not use them, ever, to throw out a remedy; although they afford a strong reason for the exhibition of a remedy that has been known to produce and cure them, in cases where there is nothing in the generals to contradict. They are often invaluable in giving the casting vote.

There may however be no marked mental symptoms, but the patient may be a very chilly patient, completely intolerant of cold. In such a case you may often reduce your work by eliminating from each rubric the hot remedies, intolerant of heat, as you work down your list. Conversely, if the patient is a hot person and intolerant of heat in every form, then only the hot remedies in each rubric need to be considered; you can disregard the chilly ones. But to be safely used, such symptoms must be general to the patient as a whole and not particular to some part (for general and particular symptoms are often contradictory), and they must be very marked. If too lightly used, there is always the risk of throwing out the remedy you need from the very start. It is this dread of missing the remedy that leads some of us to expend such an enormous amount of labour on our cases, and to use methods that Kent describes as 'hard and arduous, entailing an enormously larger amount of work than he does in his cases.' He stigmatises this as 'working uphill'.

Kent has an additional and smaller rubric of remedies affected by both heat and cold, useful where patients are intolerant of both extremes of temperature. There are both hot and cold remedies in this list.

Here I insert a list of grades, as we more or less understand them; for Kent says, 'The student and physician must strive to settle the generals, common symptoms and particulars to the fullest extent, if he wants to save work.' And a realisation of the relative importance of the marked symptoms of a case is essential for the best and quickest work.

Mentals
Will; with loves, hates fears.
Understanding; with delusions, delirium.
Memory.

Strange, Rare and Peculiar
These may occur among Mentals, Generals or Particulars, and must therefore be of varying importance and rank.

Physical
Sexual perversions (loves and hates, physical); those referred to the stomach (such as desires and aversions for foods); hot and cold foods and drinks; appetite; thirst.

Physical Generals – reactions to:
Heat and cold.
Time.
Damp and dry.
Electricity.
Oxygen and carbon dioxide.
Menstruation.
Position, gravitation.
Pressure, motion, with train-sickness, etc.
Food aggravations and ameliorations.

Character of Discharges

Particulars
These relate to a part and not the whole, and are always qualified. Kent says of them, 'Do not expect that a remedy which has the generals must also have all the little symptoms. It is a waste of time to run out all the little symptoms if the remedy has the generals. Nothing disturbs me so much as the long letters I get from doctors who show how they have wasted time on useless particulars. Common particulars are generally worthless. Get the strong, strange, peculiar symptoms, and then see to it that there are no generals in the case that oppose or contradict.'

He also says, 'When looking over a list of symptoms, first of all discover three, four, or five or six (or as many as may exist) symptoms that are strange, rare and peculiar, and work these out first. They will be the highest generals, because strange, rare and peculiar must apply to the patient himself. When you have settled upon three, four, five or six remedies that have these first generals, then find out which one of them is most like the rest of the symptoms, common and particular.'

'When you have taken a case on paper, you must next settle upon the symptoms that cannot be omitted in each individual. If he is worse from motion, you must not omit that – unless it is common, which means if it is due to inflammation. (Every inflamed and swollen joint is worse from motion, so in that case aggravation from motion is not worth much.) She is worse from consolation, hates her mother, hates her children, is worse from music, is sad before the menses, is chilly during menses, during stool, during urination. Or she is always too warm, worse in a warm room, craves cool air, all symptoms come on when she is dressed too warmly. Then see how many remedies you have; perhaps only three or four, perhaps only one. Notice whether there is anything in the case that opposes this one. If there is nothing, then give it. If you see the keynotes of Arsenicum, confirm that the patient is chilly, sensitive to air, fearful, restless, weak, pale, must have the pictures on the wall hung straight, and Arsenicum will cure.'

'Or if the keynotes look like Pulsatilla, confirm that she is not chilly, that she likes the windows open, wants to walk in the open air, is better from motion, tearful, gentle . . . To repeat: The great trouble with keynotes is that they are misused. The keynotes are often characteristic symptoms; but if the keynotes are taken as final, and the generals do not conform, then will come the failures.'

Now to the Repertory. We know what we want; let us see where to find it.

In the Repertory it is a question of the beginning and the end – the Mentals, which are in the first section of the book, and the Generalities (or Generals), which are in the final section. These are the two which are most important to us. Many a chronic case may be worked out on mentals and generals only, and the particulars will be found to fit in, in a marvellous way.

Observe that the same arrangement holds in the Mentals at the beginning, in the Generals at the end, and in all the intermediate sections. We can master it once and for all.

First, *Time*.
Next, *Conditions in alphabetical order*.
Then, when it is a question of pain, *Locality, Character, Extension*.

Take a mental symptom from the first section of the book; for example, anxiety.

First, always: Time . . . Anxiety; morning, afternoon, at night; at some special hour.

Then: Conditions under which anxiety has been observed, in alphabetical order . . . Anxiety; in open air; in bed; as of a guilty conscience; during fever; for others; before menses; about salvation; on waking, and so on.

Now turn to the last section of the Repertory – the Generalities, or Generals. Here we have the aggravations, ameliorations and reactions of the patient as a whole to his physical environment; and here again exactly the same arrangement is found.

First, in regard to Time. The patient is generally worse in the morning, at noon, at night, at such an hour. (Where no modality is specified, aggravation is always understood. 'On waking' means worse on waking. It is normal to be ameliorated by sleep. We do not repertorise the normal.)

Then, after time, come the General Conditions of the patient, as a whole, in alphabetical order. These always apply to the patient generally. (The aggravations of his various parts, head, skin, stomach, limbs, occur earlier in the book, each in its own section.)

Among these Generalities at the end of the book we find worse and better from bath and washing; from cold; from wet and dry; from position, motion, pressure, eating, sleep, and so on.

Here also, inserted alphabetically among the rest, you will find nearly all that there is of pathology in the book, and that is not much. Also certain conditions, in their alphabetical place, such as faintness; convulsions; fullness; pain in general – its onset, gradual or sudden; and its disappearance in the same way, and their combinations; its character, burning, pressing, shooting etc.; and its direction, pains that shoot up, down, inwards, outwards, across. (Elsewhere, under different headings and in their different sections, we must look for particular pains, located in head, limb, joint or organ.)

Under these broader headings, such as faintness or convulsions, you will again find qualifications, aggravations and ameliorations; and in all of these, down to the smallest sub-sections, the same order holds good. Time first, then Conditions, alphabetically. (Such as faintness morning; after midnight; at such an hour; during fever; before or after eating; on exertion; after menses; while standing, and a host of others.)

But there are also a few Generals scattered through the earlier sections of the book, and we must know where to look for them.

Desires and aversions in regard to foods are to be found in the section Stomach, with hunger and thirst – these latter with their modifications and qualifications in regard to time, first, and the other conditions in alphabetical order. Note that while hunger and thirst, and desires and aversions for different articles of diet, are placed in the section Stomach, the aggravations and ameliorations from eating, drinking, and from different kinds of food and drink are found (most of them under the heading Food) among the Generals at the end of the book.

In the same way, while the general aggravations and ameliorations in regard to the menstrual function are placed in Generalities, all the important menstrual conditions are to be found in the section Genitalia – Female. However, particulars with menstrual modifications will be found scattered from end to end in the book – for instance, various mental states modified by menses are given under their headings in the Mental section. Various headaches modified by menses are in the section Head. Stomach or abdominal distresses modified by menses are in the section Stomach or Abdomen.

Everywhere and in everything the same arrangement holds. The better and worse of the patient as a whole occurs always under Generalities. The better or worse of a part or organ (the particular) is always found in its appropriate place, such as under Head, Stomach, Chest, Extremities.

Between the Mentals at the beginning and the Generals at the end, the intermediate bulk of the book, with these few exceptions, is concerned with Particulars. That is to say, not with the patient as a whole, but with his various parts.

Let us now take pain in the extremities, the most alarming and bewildering of all the sections. It occupies more than 120 pages of the book and is not usable without knowledge of the arrangement.

It starts, as usual, with what is more general . . . pain generally in the extremities. First as to time, then the usual modifying conditions in alphabetical order, such as: during chill; when lying; during menses; rheumatic; alternating with different ailments; wandering and shifting; in wet weather, and so on.

Next, pain, as localised generally: in bones, flexor muscles; joints, nails, tendons – always qualified as to various conditions, first as regards time, and the rest in alphabetical order.

Then pain as localised in the upper limbs generally: right; left; with the same conditions following; first as to time, then the rest alphabetically; then extension.

After finishing the upper limb as a whole, Kent now takes its parts: shoulder, upper arm, elbow, forearm, wrist, hand, fingers, with all their details, to individual fingers, with joints, nails, tips; each time with conditions in the same order – time, other conditions alphabetically, then extension.

The upper limbs so far disposed of, the lower limbs are now taken in exactly the same way, with the same detail and the same arrangement; and that ends localities generally. Kent next considers the character of the pain; and under the various headings, aching, burning, cutting, drawing, etc., the whole thing is gone into again. As for instance:

Aching, generally, with its time and other conditions.

Aching in bones, joints, extensors, flexors.

Aching in upper limbs, with time, other conditions, extension.

Then aching in all the localities, in order, first of upper limb, then of lower, in each case with the usual conditions, first as to time, then the rest in alphabetical order, then extension.

So through all the various kinds of pain, burning, pressing, shooting, tearing. Each is carried down through all the localities, from the larger and more general to the smaller and more particular; and as always, with time aggravations, other conditional aggravations, and extension. Truly an amazing work.

In this way we are made free of the Repertory; for wherever Pain occurs, whether in head, stomach, bladder or back, the arrangement is the same:

First, pain generally, in regard to time and other conditions – these always in alphabetical order.

Next, pain localised, in regard to time; other conditions; extension.

Then character of pain generally, with time; other conditions; extension.

Then character of pain in regard to each locality in turn, always with regard to time; other conditions in alphabetical order; extension.

The homoeopath is already familiar with the broader arrangement of the Repertory, for it is that of the Materia Medica. Let us just glance through it, as there are a few points of difficulty in the search for what we want. Taking the sections in order:

Mentals. Here especially we need to read constantly, and compare. We may often have to take the idea and resort to synonyms in order to find just what we need. Sometimes we have to combine rubrics. Among the Mentals, the sub-sections are often far more important than the lists under the large and more general headings. Weeping is a very long rubric and is common to very many remedies. It is qualified, for example, by weeping at a certain hour; alternating with cheerfulness; causeless; consolation aggravates; while telling symptoms; from music. These things individualise and carry us nearer to the remedy. It repays you to constantly study the Mentals; to know exactly what you can find there, and under what precise phraseology. Observe that sensitive to light, noise, etc., are here; while sensitive to odours comes under 'Smell, acute', in the section *Nose*.

Vertigo. Here are several headings that denote levitation; sensations of sinking; tendency to fall to right, left, etc.

Head. Includes hair. Here we get all the head sensations and pains; and here, for head only, we get what we had previously noted in Generalities for pain generally, i.e. increasing and decreasing, suddenly or gradually, and their combinations.

Eye. With a separate section, *Vision*.

Ear. With discharges and pains, but with a separate section, *Hearing*.

Nose, including its function, Smell.

Face.

Mouth, including Tongue, which is interwoven into all its sections; but with a separate section for *Teeth*. (Coated tongue is found under 'Mouth, discolouration'.)

From mouth, away down the digestive tube, taking first *Throat*, with tonsils, uvula, oesophagus. Kent then inserts *External Throat*, with cervical glands and thyroid. This section is always difficult to find.

Stomach, with the important generals – the desires and aversions in regard to articles of diet, hunger and thirst. (As mentioned already, better and worse for eating and drinking, and for different foods, are found in *Generalities*.)

Abdomen. Here most of the menstrual pains are to be found. As it is often difficult to differentiate between gastric and abdominal pain, it is advisable to consult both these sections.

Rectum, with a separate section for *Stool*. Diarrhoea, constipation and urging are found under *Rectum*, whereas character of stool – loose, hard, large, gushing, forcible, colour, odour, etc. are under *Stool*.

Then under *Urinary Organs* we get no less than five sections. They are puzzling at first, because Bladder and Urine are widely separated and one hardly knows what to look for in each. These sections are: *Bladder*, *Kidneys*, *Prostate Gland*, *Urethra*, *Urine*. Urging, retention, etc. occur under Bladder; whereas the character of the urine, its odour and deposits are to be found under Urine. Here also we find Urine, copious and scanty.

Genitalia, in two sections, for *Male* and *Female*. In the latter are the important generals associated with menstruation, whereas the generally worse and better in connection with menses are under *Generalities*, at the end of the book.

Then we are taken back to the throat, to start this time down the respiratory tract. Kent's order in compiling the Repertory is always: from above, down; from the more important to the less; from the most broadly general to the most minutely particular:

Larynx and Trachea.

Respiration.

Cough.

Expectoration.

Then *Chest*, into whose sections are interwoven lungs, heart, mammae.

Back.

Extremities.

Next, *Sleep*, with dreams. Really an important general. This includes positions in sleep; whereas better and worse for sleep, and for different positions lying, are found at the end of the book in *Generalities*.

Then the Fever sections . . . *Chill, Fever, Perspiration.* (Under *Fever*, you find the succession, or stages, which may be important.)

Then *Skin*; which, remember, is merely a particular, an organ, though a very important one as regards its excretory function.

The book concludes with the all-important section, *Generalities*.

Remedy Index

Page numbers in bold type refer to a full remedy picture in Section III of this book.

281

Subject Index

Classical Homoeopathy, Dr Margery Blackie, 1986, reprinted 1990 with Repertory. The complete teaching legacy of one of the most important homoeopaths of our time. 0906584140

Comparative Materia Medica, Dr E. F. Candegabe, 1997. Detailed comparative study of thirty-seven remedies by one of the Argentinian masters. 0906584361

Everyday Homoeopathy (2nd Edition), Dr David Gemmell, 1997. A practical handbook for using homoeopathy in the context of one's own personal and family health care, using readily available remedies. 0906584442

Homoeopathic Prescribing, Dr Noel Pratt, revised 1985. A compact reference book covering 161 common complaints and disorders, with guidance on the choice of the appropriate remedy. 0906584035

Homoeopathic Treatment of Beef and Dairy Cattle, The, C. E. I. Day, MRCVS, 1995. Describes how homoeopathy may be used in the care of cattle, both as individuals and in a group. 090658437X

Homoeopathic Treatment of Eczema, Robin Logan, FSHom (in preparation). A textbook on the homoeopathic treatment of this condition. 0906584477

Homoeopathy, Dr T. P. Paschero (in preparation). Dr Paschero's major work on the subject. 0906584418

Homoeopathy as Art and Science, Dr Elizabeth Wright Hubbard, 1990. The selected writings of one of the foremost modern homoeopaths. 0906584264

Homoeopathy in Practice, Dr Douglas Borland, 1982, reprinted 1988 with Symptom Index. Detailed guidance on the observation of symptoms and the choice of remedies. 090658406X

In Search of the Later Hahnemann, Rima Handley, DPhil, FSHom, 1997. A study of Hahnemann's practice in Paris, with material from his casebooks of that period. 0906584353

Insights into Homoeopathy, Dr Frank Bodman, 1990. Homoeopathic approaches to common problems in general medicine and psychiatry. 0906584280

Introduction to Homoeopathic Medicine (2nd Edition), Dr Hamish Boyd, 1989. A formal introductory text, written in categories that are familiar to the medical practitioner. 0906584213

Materia Medica of New Homoeopathic Remedies, Dr O. A. Julian, paperback edition 1984. Full clinical coverage of 106 new homoeopathic remedies, for use in conjunction with the classical materia medicas.   0906584116

Mental Symptoms in Homoeopathy, Dr Luis Detinis, 1994. A comparative study of the Mind rubrics in Kent's *Repertory*.   0906584345

Studies of Homoeopathic Remedies, Dr Douglas Gibson, 1987. Detailed clinical studies of 100 major remedies. Well-known for the uniquely wide range of insights brought to bear on each remedy.
0906584175

Tutorials on Homoeopathy, Dr Donald Foubister, 1989. Detailed studies on a wide range of conditions and remedies.   0906584256

Typology in Homoeopathy, Dr Léon Vannier, 1992. A study of human types, based on the gods of Antiquity, and the remedies which are relevant to them.   0906584302